BREASTFEEDING, NURSING AND JUST PLAIN UDDERANCE

THE GIRLFRIEND'S GUIDE TO BREASTFEEDING

HEATHER DE PAULO

This book is for anyone who is having a baby and would like to provide human milk for their babies, regardless of gender, sexual orientation, race or religion.

Copyright © 2021 Heather de Paulo
All rights reserved.

First edition September 2021

ISBN 978-1-7374077-0-6 (ebook)
ISBN 978-1-7374077-1-3 (paperback)

www.heathermichellenutritionist.com

This book is dedicated to all my girlfriends who supported me, encouraged me, opened up and told me their personal stories to help others, provided me with real, honest feedback, and gave me the confidence to write this book.

Contents

Part I - Ready to Pop 1

Chapter 1 - Getting the Right Mindset 3
Get the Right Mindset from the Start 4
Choosing your Birthing Team 7

Chapter 2 - The Baby is Born Now What? 8
What Happens if Baby Still Won't Latch On? 9
How Do You Know You're Getting a Good Latch? 10
What Do I Do with Flat Nipples? 12
What is Baby Actually Getting? 12

Part II - The First Two Weeks 15

Chapter 3 - Home with Baby 17
The Reality of Getting Started 18
You Have Enough Milk! 20
Augmented Breasts 22
How Often Will My Baby Feed? 23
Only Milk Needed 24

  Cracked Nipple Prevention 25

  Feeding Comfortably 26

  Help in the First Weeks 27

 Chapter 4 - Oh, Those Visitors! 29

Part III - The One Year Stint 33

 Chapter 5 - Getting Out There 35

  Peer Pressure 38

  Aren't Babies Supposed to Be Chunky? 39

  Human Pacifier 41

  When Can I Start My Baby on the Bottle? 41

 Chapter 6 - Other Stuff You Should Know 41

  Yikes, My Baby Doesn't Want the Breast Anymore! 42

  Ouch! Does He Have Teeth Already? 43

  No, I Didn't Pee My Shirt 43

  Clogged Ducts and Mastitis 45

  I'm Dying for a Glass of Wine 47

  Breasts are for Feeding, not for Sex! 49

  Nine-Month Slump 50

 Chapter 7 - Getting Back to Work 52

  Now I Really Feel Like a Cow! 54

  Storing Milk 57

  Can I Mix Milk? 58

  What Happened to My Milk? 60

Part IV - Nutrition 65

 Chapter 8 - What Do I Need and How Much? 67

  Vitamin D 68

  Omega-3s 68

  Calcium 70

  Protein 71

  Fluids 72

Chapter 9 - Giving Up Your Favorite Foods – is it Necessary? 74

Chapter 10 - Herbs – What Should You Know? 79

  Herbs That May Boost Supply 80

  Herbs That May Decrease Supply 81

Chapter 11 - Weight Loss – or Gain? 84

  Not Rockin' Your High School Jeans? 84

  Why the Weight isn't Melting Off – Nerd Out Section 85

  The Good News 88

  The Big Secret 89

Part V - After One Year 93

Chapter 12 - Your Baby is a Year Old! What's Next? 95

  Which type of Milk is Best? 95

  No Periods Yet? 96

  Still Not Sleeping Through the Night? 97

  Grabbing the Boob in Public 98

Epilogue 100

Resources 103

Author Note 113

About the Author 116

Preface

Breastfeeding is one of the most amazing things we women have the unique ability to do. Besides actually being pregnant and feeling your baby growing in your belly, providing magic milk for your newborn is something only you can do, and it's something truly remarkable. You will cherish those moments when it's just you and your baby, when he or she looks up at you, strokes your chest, or reaches up and touches your face while feeding. Mommy and me time at its finest! You will never experience anything like it, and it passes by in the blink of an eye.

I decided early on, even before pregnancy, that I was going to breastfeed my babies. Once I got pregnant, I worked on creating the mindset that I would be successful at it. I read up the wazoo about everything baby-related – pregnancy, labor and delivery, and, of course, breastfeeding. I had some challenges along the way, but once I got past the first couple of weeks, it was (mostly) smooth sailing – no leaking, no bleeding or cracking, and perfect, not huge, breasts (I miss those breasts!). Though I did experience clogged ducts a few times (which isn't fun), I really have to say that, overall, I had a great breastfeeding experience with both of my babies that I will cherish forever. I do chalk much of my success up to my mindset, which is what I want to pass on to you in this book.

A couple of years ago, I had what you may call a "premonition" to write this book: What to write, the sections, the title, what the book cover would look like – everything came to me very vividly. But I sat on it and didn't do anything. More recently, I started to do some self-reflection and in the midst of it, the idea of the book came to me again. I thought, "This must be a sign. I cannot ignore it this time; I HAVE to write this book!" I started thinking about all the women out there who I could help with my insight and experience, so I just sat down and started typing.

Initially, I thought it was going to be a sort of booklet, a quick read, maybe 20 to 30 pages of some encouragement and tips to help you, the soon-to-be mother, or the mother struggling with the whole breastfeeding thing, to be successful in your breastfeeding journey. But, as time went on, and I started talking to other women about their trials and tribulations, as well as reading questions women had, I kept adding and adding. Plus, since I'm a registered dietitian, so I thought I should include a chapter on nutrition, right?

Over the years, I have spoken to and read comments from women who didn't have such a great journey. They really struggled with breastfeeding their babies for numerous reasons. Therefore, I decided to interview girlfriends, some who had great experiences, to tap into what worked for them, and some that didn't, so each of you can relate, learn, be successful in your efforts, and know you aren't the only one out there experiencing the exact same thing! I included stories and tips from some of these women so that you can perhaps identify with them, and hopefully their experiences will help you deal with any issues you may be having.

This book is written in a "girlfriend to girlfriend" style. Imagine that we are BFFs. I've successfully breastfed my babies, you are preggo and are asking for advice on breastfeeding. We are sitting over a coffee, a virgin daiquiri (because you're pregnant), or whatever your fav beverage is. We are lounging on a sofa, in a lounge chair by the pool or on the beach, by the fire, or wherever else you fancy, and I'm giving you my best advice because I love you as a sister. When you read this book, that's how I want you to visualize it!

There may be some redundancy, but redundancy is good because then the information really sticks! Plus, maybe you are one of those people who skip around or your mind drifts while reading, so I want to make sure you don't miss anything!

This is by no means an all-inclusive book. If it was, it would probably be more than 1000 pages long, and I really wanted it to be a book that is a quick read, that you find doable, not a long book that seems overwhelming. I added the key points that I think are crucial to developing the right mindset to be successful, and some extra information and advice on questions I saw repeatedly from new moms. I have a lot of additional information to supplement the book that you can get via my resource booklet; my gift to you as one of my readers! Check it out at **www.heathermichellenutritionist.com/resourcebooklet**.

When I started this book, I was giving blanket recommendations for things that I loved when I was breastfeeding, but then I thought, "why not make your life easier?" I've already done the research, so I've included a resources section on my website with products I love at **www.heathermichellenutritionist.com/goodies**. All you have to do is click and find what you need, no searching around looking for stuff.

One more thing to add. I'm focused on exclusively giving breast milk, primarily via the breast, but however you can give it. I'm not judging anyone, and you have to do what you feel you have to do, but don't send me hate mail because I'm expressing my opinion that the breast is best and you should only resort to formula as a last resort. I want you to know where this book is going from the get-go. But also know that most women who turn to formula do so because they don't have the proper support. That's the whole purpose of this book – to empower you and help you set yourself up, not only with the right mindset, but to really get prepared to be successful at breastfeeding.

Think about it, have you really done anything truly important in your life without preparing? I think the only amazing thing we can do without preparing in one way or another is actually conceiving. Your education, your job, any other major accomplishments in your life – did you just sit back, let them happen and you were successful at accomplishing them and accomplishing them well? If you did, please contact me immediately because I want to hear your story; it will be some kind of miracle!

I'm neither a doctor nor a certified lactation consultant; I'm a registered dietitian and a mom with quite some years of experience. If you are ever in doubt about something, please consult the appropriate professional. There are many resources to help you out there. You can find some resources in the appendix of this book.

Finally, no blanket recommendation or method will work for absolutely everyone because we are human beings, individuals, and we all think and react differently to things. Just because I may mention that getting started is difficult or it hurts, doesn't mean it will be for you. While I want to prepare you for what you may experience, you may breeze right on through, so don't assume that you will have the same experience as others. Also, you will find that many times I mention that you will have to try things out yourself to see if they work for you. This is why. There's a lot of trial and error in this process, so you just need to have confidence in the gift Mother Nature gave you to produce milk for your baby, and the patience to find what works best for you.

It is my sincere wish that this book empowers you to have confidence in your ability to breastfeed your baby. Without further delay, let's get started on this journey together!

Part I
Ready to Pop

To be or not to be… that was what Hamlet asked, but for ladies in our day and age, preparing to give birth to a miracle, the question is: *To breastfeed or not to breastfeed?*

Chapter 1
Getting the Right Mindset

Since you are my BFF, I'm going to share a secret with you. I gave my babies something that fights off viruses and bacteria, lowers the risk of not only colds and infections, but asthma, allergies, sudden infant death syndrome (SIDS), respiratory infections, gut infections, diabetes, dental problems, and is also the perfect nutrition for babies. Not only is it so amazing for your baby, you benefit as well! It helps you burn calories, helps your uterus contract back to normal, gives you some relief from having your period (some ladies, longer than others), lowers your risk of breast and ovarian cancers and also osteoporosis. Would you pull out your credit card on the spot to ask me to get you some immediately?

What if I told you it's free? You may just have to work a little bit to get it, particularly in the beginning, but once you get over the hump, it's (mostly) smooth sailing! It's just like when you start working out again after being on hiatus for a while. You suffer through the workouts and are sore as hell for a few weeks, but then it gets easier and more and more enjoyable, and you love the results you get!

Of course, you know I'm talking about breast milk! I'm sure you've heard all of these benefits for you and the baby before (if not, I have a whole list in my resource booklet at **www.heathermichellenutritionist.com/resourcebooklet**). However, if it's such a no-brainer, then why do so few women choose to breastfeed or don't stick with it very long? Well, besides not getting the education, support, or being in the right social environment for success, it's just plain hard to get started. I mean, here you are, with a new baby, totally overwhelmed [this baby is YOURS, and you (and your partner) are solely responsible for it], and now you have to try to get this screaming, hungry baby to latch on properly to your boob. What does that even mean, "latch on properly?" And it freaking HURTS! On top of it all, you have your nurse, pediatrician, or mother-in-law (or all three) taunting you with a can of formula, tempting you with the easy way out.

Since I mentioned formula, I just want to say a couple of things. Again no guilt here, just facts. First of all, when you breastfeed, think about the money and hassle you save. Formula is freaking expensive! Doing a little research, you can spend anywhere from $1000 to $3000 a year on formula, depending on which type of formula you use. Not to mention all of the bottles, nipples, sterilizing equipment, and so on. If cost doesn't matter much to you, what about when your baby is screaming in a restaurant or on an airplane and you have to get out all the stuff and mix the formula, hoping the water is at the right temperature, with people giving you dirty looks like, "why doesn't she just shut that baby up?".

If that still doesn't convince you, just take a look at the ingredients label. Most formulas have mostly powdered cow milk, whey protein solids, and various vegetable oils, then a bunch of vitamins and minerals and other things they add to try to mimic breast milk. Some formulas have corn syrup solids and sugar listed in the top 5 ingredients! Organic formula is better, you say? How about organic nonfat milk, organic corn maltodextrin, organic sugar, organic high oleic sunflower oil, etc. Does it sound better because it says organic? At least the first ingredient is not corn syrup, but milk in most formulas comes from cows. Do you think your human baby will do better drinking processed cow milk with sugar and oils (and added synthetic vitamins and minerals), or the milk your body makes solely to meet the specific nutrient needs for your bundle of joy? OK, I'm off my soapbox about formula, but I hope you get what I mean.

Get the Right Mindset from the Start

No matter if this is your first pregnancy or your fifth (and you didn't breastfeed the others or struggled with the others and just don't want to deal with it again), it's never too late to get the right mindset to give your baby the best of what nature has to offer. The first thing you have to do is make up your mind that you will only give your precious baby mother's milk!! There is no "try." It's not something you try, it's something you DO. Like Yoda says, "Do or do not; there is no try." This is one of the best pieces of advice ever in life, and especially in breastfeeding because you are pretty much guaranteed to have challenges. If you are one of those women in the try mindset, I'm glad you picked up my book! That means that you are interested in educating yourself on breastfeeding and developing the right mindset to be successful!

My friend Lanie, who has five children, had the right mindset:

> *You have to be determined in knowing that this (breastfeeding) is the best for your child in order to work through the difficulties and not give up.*

Besides the challenges of just getting started, you will encounter many naysayers on the way. "I never breastfed my baby and he is just fine." "I didn't have enough milk, so I couldn't breastfeed my baby." "Your baby is so skinny/crying/not sleeping through the night, you must not have enough milk." "Your baby is premature, so you will have to supplement with formula." The latter happened to me. I recognize that, depending on the amount of prematurity, some babies will definitely need to be supplemented with formula, but my daughter (my second born) was born exactly a month early and, thankfully, she didn't have to go into the NICU (Neonatal Intensive Care Unit). I got up to pee one night and liquid kept pouring out of me – I couldn't make it stop! I realized then that it wasn't pee – my water broke! I wasn't ready – you can imagine the chaos in my house in the wee hours of the morning, trying to pack the hospital bag, and rushing off to the hospital! Then, within 45 minutes of getting super-intense labor pains, she was out! A few hours later, the OB and pediatrician both told me, "You will have to supplement her with formula." Because my mind was made up to give only breast milk, my thought was, no way I'm giving my baby formula! And my daughter grew just fine, gaining weight in no time! I won't lie to you, it was challenging, but my mind was made up and I was confident in my decision. You need to be confident too!

My friend Kim had it right:

> *If you think there's an alternative, you won't make it. I had a goal W of breastfeeding for six months and didn't even think of alternatives.*

A way to gain confidence is to educate yourself – read, read, read! I can tell you there are NO books that will tell you formula is better than breastfeeding. Even some formula cans tell you breast milk is better. If you arm yourself with knowledge on WHY you are choosing to breastfeed and prepare yourself to give an educated response to the negative comments of the naysayers, you will be ready and it will give you the confidence you need to persevere. I've had to do this more than once, even pulling out my books and literally showing references to support what I was doing (i.e. to the questioning mother-in-law!). This is what my friend Kathleen had to say about her experience:

> *I had a lot of trouble with blocked ducts with all three of my babies. It was very painful. And my first wouldn't latch on, there was nothing natural about it. My husband was frustrated and wanted to buy formula. He was afraid our son was starving and wasn't getting enough nutrition. I was lucky to have support from a lactation specialist; if not, I would have given up. What helped me persevere is that I read and educated myself on the importance of breastfeeding. All of the books said that breastfeeding is the best option.*

By the way, your husband, significant other, or friend who's helping you needs to be on board with you 100%, so include him or her in the education process. You need to know he or she will support you when you are doubting yourself, when meddling in-laws try to tell you that you should just use formula, and when you just don't feel sexy (more about that later!).

I want to speak to those of you for whom this isn't your first go around. Perhaps this is your second baby or your third, and you were previously unsuccessful. Maybe that's why you picked up this book – because you have the desire and just need some help and support. No worries, you came to the right place! You can make this work! Whatever happened to you before is not guaranteed to happen again. The only guarantee you have of a repeat is staying with the same mindset you had before. Remember, if you do what you always did, you will get what you always got. Take my advice – change your mindset, educate yourself, and surround yourself with supportive people. Better yet, have people around you who have gone through it and know how to really help you. Have everything set up BEFORE the birth. This will pay off exponentially!

Choosing your Birthing Team

When you are choosing your doctor, you need to make sure that he or she, and your whole birthing team, is on the same page as you and will respect your wishes. At the moment of giving birth, you won't be thinking straight and will need someone who will expedite your plan. A doctor is just a person and they aren't doing this for free. They are getting paid a lot of money, so you need to interview your doctor just as you would interview a person for one of the most important positions in your life. And if one doctor doesn't click, move on to another one! We all know that doctors don't have all day to sit with you and answer 100 questions, but be organized and efficient and have your list of questions ready when you have your appointments. If your doctor rolls his eyes or she always seems like she's trying to get out of the room with a hand on the doorknob, move on to another doctor. And don't get pressured by your friends who say Dr. XYZ is "the best" OB in town. That OB may be the best for them, but not you.

You also need a birthing plan so everyone knows what you want and what you expect from them during and after the labor and delivery process. The hospital where I gave birth was known to stick a bottle in the baby's mouth, even when the mother expressed the desire to breastfeed. I made sure my plan was very clear that this WAS NOT to happen, and that I wanted my baby with me at all times! It is VERY important to make sure you have a team that will support your decision to exclusively breastfeed your baby. Once a baby gets an artificial nipple, it will be more challenging to get him to latch on to your breast. Artificial is much easier, the formula comes pouring out. A baby has to work harder to get milk out of a breast. So, it's very important to make sure that your baby's first experience with getting milk is from the breast (of course, there are exceptions, like with premature babies).

Now, let me just say here that if, for whatever reason, your baby gets a bottle before your breast, don't throw in the towel and think it's too late to breastfeed. Of course, many babies latch on to a breast after having a bottle, so all is not lost. It just may be a little more challenging, but definitely doable! I'm just saying, why not set yourself up for the path of least resistance from the get-go?

Chapter 2
The Baby is Born! Now What?

You just went through a (probably) painful, natural labor, or a C-section and are strapped to a table, or you just went through a painful labor AND a C-section and now you have this beautiful baby. Now what? The last thing you may be thinking of at that moment is to put the baby on your breast, but that's exactly what you need to do. As soon as the baby is out, don't let the nurses whisk him off to weigh, clean, poke and prod. You need to make sure you make it very clear to your doctor and your team that you want your baby immediately on your breast (unless there's a medical reason why this isn't possible). This is why it's so important to choose your team wisely and make sure you have your birth plan ready beforehand. Maybe there's a new person in the room who didn't see your birthing plan (like, if you happen to be so lucky as to give birth on Labor Day when you have a skeleton crew at the hospital). You or your significant other need to make sure your wishes are carried out. DO NOT get intimidated! This is YOUR baby and you have a right to have your wishes met!

I will tell you that it's likely that the baby will not latch on right away. Neither of my babies did. When it's your first baby, it feels weird to try to stick your nipple in baby's mouth. But the act of it, and getting baby close to you so he can smell mama right away, is good enough to get things started. After that point, you can let the team take your baby to do what they are itching to do, and after you get cleaned up, stitched up (if needed), and get a much, much needed drink of something cold, you can get comfortable in your room and try again.

What Happens if Baby Still Won't Latch On?

You are cleaned up, stitched up, comfy (as you can be) in your room, baby in your arms, admiring your perfect bundle of joy, checking all ten fingers and toes, discussing with your significant other who's nose she has – the perfect moment (or maybe not, but work with me here). You decide it's time to try to get the baby to latch on again. It's nature, right? Baby should just know what to do, right? But, as you awkwardly try to put your nipple in baby's mouth, it doesn't happen. Your baby doesn't seem interested or doesn't quite seem to get the nipple in. Maybe you have huge nipples and you wonder how they will get in that tiny mouth? In this tranquil setting, (aahhh so sweet) you decide to just wait a little while longer and try again.

That is the calm, cool and collected scenario. How about a different scenario? The baby is screaming. You are stressed, hubby is stressed, baby isn't latching on, you are freaking out that baby is hungry, you start doubting yourself and your ability to breastfeed your baby. You call a nurse to come help, she tries to help, but it's still not working. She gives you the look – "why not just give your baby formula – it's easier." NOOOOO! Do not succumb!

Babies cry – get used to it. They have no way to communicate, so they cry. They cry when they are hungry, but they also cry when they have a dirty diaper, they cry when they are cold, they cry when they are hot, they cry when they are tired, they cry when they want to be held, they cry for just about everything. You will get to know the cries and what they mean as time goes on, but for now, it's important to know that your baby won't starve to death if he doesn't get milk immediately. In fact, babies can take a few days after birth before they start eating properly, so don't fear. You have plenty of time to get the hang of it. Keep in mind that if you needed any medications during your labor, they affect the baby too. Their little livers don't metabolize drugs very well, so they may be extra sleepy and not interested in eating for a day or so. Of course, when in doubt, ask your doctor or midwife. Since you already did your homework to choose one who understands your dedication to breastfeeding, he or she will steer you in the right direction.

How Do You Know You're Getting a Good Latch?

OK, so telling you in writing won't really replace someone actually helping you in person, but it might at least help you get an idea of what a good latch should look like. My friend Michelle jokingly said it's when your Cuban grandmother thinks you are suffocating the baby! All joking aside, if you feel like your baby isn't latching well, or if you are really having excruciating pain when trying to feed, look to see that you have the following going on:

- Baby's chin should be tucked into your breast, and his or her mouth should be wide open with the bottom lip curled back.
- Baby's nose will be clear or only just be touching your breast.
- More of your areola will be visible above your baby's top lip than below it.
- Baby's cheeks should not be sucking in and there should be no clicking noise during sucking.
- There should be no nipple pain — but you might feel a stretching sensation as your nipple adjusts to breastfeeding. Ha, this one is wishful thinking. I'm sorry to tell you, but you will have nipple pain in the beginning. I mean, maybe you've had one of those crazy sex weekends with a boob man who was on them constantly, but nothing compares to a baby sucking on those nipples every couple of hours. It WILL hurt in the first couple of weeks, so be ready for it. After a couple of weeks, the pain will go away and you won't feel anything, as long as you have the right latch.

OK, it may take longer for some women. My friend, Kim, said it took three months before things went smoothly with no issues. Here's what my friend Denise said:

> I had a rough time with my daughter. Every time she would latch on, I would have to grab a pillow. It took a month to six weeks before the pain subsided. Looking back, she probably wasn't latching right. The pain probably went away because I was finally able to get a good latch.

If you are still having pain after two weeks, check to make sure you have a good latch or rule out anything else that may have an identifiable solution (like a tongue tie). For those of you who just take longer, you must keep in mind your "why," like my friend Kathleen did. Why are you choosing to breastfeed? Because it's the best thing you can give your baby.

My friend Michelle had twins born at 30 weeks and they spent 40 days in the NICU (Neonatal Intensive Care Unit):

> *I couldn't get my babies on the breast for over a month; I just pumped 10 times a day to keep up for two and give them all the breast milk I could. When I was finally able to put them on the breast, it took many days and attempts for them to get a proper latch. I did a lot of trying and learned the technique. It took me around 3-4 weeks for them to really get a good latch and feed off the breast.*

If it's really not working out for you, please find some help before you give up. In fact, get help before it even gets that far. Check out the appendix for some recommendations. If you can't afford a nurse or lactation consultant, ask a friend who's successfully breastfed her babies. Perhaps it can be your mom, like my friends Lilian and Randi.

Lilian:

> *My mother was available to help me. In her time, everyone breastfed. I'm from Singapore and formula was very expensive because everything is imported, so it wasn't an option. Shortly after I had my daughter, I moved to the US and didn't know what types of formulas I should even try, plus it was just so much easier to breastfeed than dealing with bottles during the whole moving process, so I'm grateful for my mom's help to get me on the right track early on.*

Randi:

> *I was fortunate because I had my mom as my "lactation consultant." She breastfed us at a time when breastfeeding was trending out in the early 1950s. She initially breastfed us for economic reasons, but later realized the benefits to us and also to her.*

If a friend or your mom isn't available, ask your pediatrician or OB if he or she knows someone who can help, or look up a La Leche League or Women, Infants and Children (WIC) center in your area. The point is, there's help everywhere, so seek it out – preferably before you give birth.

What Do I Do with Flat Nipples?

Some women have flat or inverted nipples – maybe you. It's absolutely false that you cannot breastfeed. There are things you can do to help get that nipple out and ready for feeding. One item that many women swear by is a latch assistant. You can find these just about anywhere. It basically has a bulb on the end of a plastic flange that goes over your nipple. When you squeeze the bulb, it sucks your nipple out, kind of like a nasal aspirator that you use to suck the snot out of a baby's nose. I know, not a pretty picture, but many things that happen with babies aren't pretty, and if it gets your nipple out, it's worth it! Another item you may hear about is breast shells – many women swear by them. They come with two types of backs: one with a bigger hole to put a barrier between your nipple and clothing when they are really sore, and one with a smaller hole that you wear in your bra to help get your nipple out. They aren't meant to be worn around all day, just for 30 minutes or so before a feeding (which sounds inconvenient, because you have to remember to put them in). Whether or not you have inverted nipples, if you are a leaker and breast pads don't really work for you, maybe you can try using breast shells.

On another note, what about using an ice cube? Do your nipples poke out when you get really cold? This may work! You can also try pumping a little first to get your nipple out. The point is that you can be very successful with inverted or flat nipples. What works or doesn't depends on the grade of inversion you have, but hang in there! If none of the techniques I mentioned work, get help from your doctor, a lactation consultant, or another resource available in your area.

What is Baby Actually Getting?

At first, your body is making colostrum, which is thick and is provided in small amounts. Colostrum has the exact nutrition your baby needs at that stage in her little life (in fact, you have probably seen supplements of colostrum on the market because it's so nutrient-rich). Then, when the time is right, in around three to five days, your milk comes in. Some women get a huge deluge, for others, their breasts get larger, but it's not like the dam broke. I had both with my babies. With my son, it was more normal, with my daughter, it was like someone filled my breasts with that stuff you put in a tire when it's flat – like BABOOM! My point is, don't freak out if you don't get the BABOOM, it doesn't mean you don't have enough milk. Your body will make what your baby needs.

When your milk does come in, that's the moment when your baby needs the calories for growth. You will see a difference in the way your baby feeds too – you will see and even hear her swallow. It's normal for babies to lose up to 10% of their birthweight shortly after birth, but within one week, your baby will typically have gained back the birth weight she lost, some may lose a little less and some a little more, but if you see your baby is gaining weight, it's good! You will also be changing more diapers and that goopy black poop (meconium) will become softer and more yellowish. These are all good signs! Of course, if you have any questions about weight, pee, and poop, ask your nurse, midwife, or doctor.

Part II
The First Two Weeks

Being home with the baby the first couple of nights can be overwhelming. It dawns on you that you are the one responsible for this baby; she's yours and you can't give her back to anyone! Just take a deep breath and be grateful for your bundle of joy. You've got this!

Chapter 3
Home with Baby

You finally get home with the baby (or maybe you gave a home birth). The crowd around the whole experience has died down and you finally have some alone time with your baby and your significant other. You are definitely going to feel overwhelmed, especially that first night alone, so just mentally prepare for it. Waking up in the middle of the night, feeling exhausted, still trying to get a hang of the breastfeeding thing, and in these first couple of weeks, it's all you because you are the provider of all of the meals. Your significant other will be able to help out with some things, but for now, you need to make sure you and your baby get a hang of this breastfeeding thing.

There are a couple of things I recommend you have for the baby – a co-sleeper and a nursing pillow. If you plan to let the baby sleep in your bed, that's up to you, but I definitely don't recommend having a whole separate crib for the baby where you have to literally get up out of bed and walk to another location to tend to the baby every time she wakes up. When you hear of parents complaining of exhaustion, this is a big part of it. I had a friend who told me she never dealt with anything so difficult in her life – and then I found out she was actually walking downstairs to her daughter's nursery several times a night to tend to her crying baby! No wonder she was so tired! Trust me, a co-sleeper is worth every penny. It's basically just an extension of your bed, so your baby is right next to you, but in his own space. When he wakes up at night, you can just roll over, pull him next to you and on the breast, and when he's done, you just place him back in his space. I won't lie, I would snooze off while he was on the breast, but when I would wake up, baby would be asleep and it was very easy to put him back in his co-sleeper. Of course, to change a diaper, you do have to sit up, but that's a lot better than walking to the other side of the room. I had a little night light so I could keep the room dark with just enough light to see what I was doing. Sometimes, my husband would talk to me in these moments and I would tell him, "I'm not really awake." Basically, don't start a conversation with me because I don't want to fully wake up!

Babies also make a lot of noise at night – grunts and small cries. With a co-sleeper, you can just roll over and open one eye to see the baby. When you see all is OK, you can just drift back off to sleep. You aren't one to fall back to sleep so easily, you say? Let me tell you, that won't be a problem at this stage in the game. Your body will take advantage of every possible chance to get some shut-eye!

The nursing pillow is great because you are going to be spending a lot of time holding your baby on your breast and believe me, those seven to ten pounds get heavy! Plus, it also allows you to free up your hands. I caught up on a lot of reading while sitting in my rocker-glider chair, baby on my breast, laying on the nursing pillow. It was really worth having one.

That reminds me – there are actually three things you need – a co-sleeper, a nursing pillow, and a rocker-glider chair WITH the rocking ottoman. You will be spending many hours in your rocker-glider; it's worth investing in a comfortable one! Check out my recommendations for all three at: **www.heathermichellenutritionist.com/goodies**.

The Reality of Getting Started

I mentioned it before, but I'm going to say it again - the first two weeks are the most difficult. It's awkward and it hurts (at least for most of us). My friend Amy said she wasn't prepared for how much it would hurt because no one told her, so I'm telling you now! Your nipples need to toughen up. Think about someone who needs to build callouses on her hands to do a new job. It hurts at first, but then the body adapts. Thankfully, your nipples will NOT build callouses, so don't freak out! But they do adapt so that you don't even feel it anymore.

First, the nipple hurts like hell when baby latches on. This is why it's very important to get a proper latch. If baby doesn't latch correctly, problems start, like pain and cracking. This is where a lactation consultant can help you get a proper latch if this is a problem. Then, while your baby is on your breast, hormones are released that tell your uterus to contract, so think severe menstrual cramps. I can understand why some women give up because it's very uncomfortable at this stage, but you have to remember the determination you built up and the education you now have in your arsenal on how this is the absolute best for your baby. Remember your WHY! Now is not the time to think about yourself and your discomfort. I promise it gets much easier!

After a few days of this, the real milk comes in and BABOOM!! Breasts you never knew you could have! Some of us are very pleased with this, you may be saying, "YES!", while others may not be so pleased and are saying, "NO!" If you get the really big BABOOM, I can tell you that in the first week or so, it does hurt or will be uncomfortable, especially when you lay on your back. Thankfully, it will subside and your breasts will become a size that you can handle with no pain.

Remember my premature daughter? The one everyone told me I would have to supplement with formula? I was absolutely determined to feed her exclusively breast milk. That girl was on my boob every freaking half an hour, 24 hours a day. It hurt like hell, and the uterus contracting felt like labor all over again. On top of that, when she would latch on, she would do this thing where she would flick my nipple with her tongue, so it felt like a knife on my already sore nipples. And when my milk came in – WOW! There are straps that go around your whole torso that you can use to literally strap your breasts down to help alleviate the pain, and I was definitely using one in those first days; I could not lay down without that strap around my chest. But, after about a week, things had already subsided and by two weeks, she was feeding at more regular intervals, the pain was gone and my breasts were down to a beautiful size. Plus, she regained her birth weight in one week and kept gaining from there. So, yes, it was hell, but it was all worth it and now I have this great story to tell!

If you are so engorged that you feel like you are going to explode, there are things you can do to alleviate the engorgement. The first thought would be to get that baby on the breast, but perhaps your breasts are so hard, she can't even latch on. To soften your breasts a bit, you can express a little with a pump, or by hand, if you are so talented. You can also try running warm water over your breasts in the shower or using a hot washcloth to loosen things up and get the milk flowing. If you are really having a lot of pain, you can even use ice packs or frozen vegetable bags to reduce swelling and discomfort. Just don't worry, this is temporary and it will pass!

Before we leave the topic of painful nipples, I want to mention one more thing. My friend Peggy shared that after her son was around four months old, she started getting pain in her nipples again. Here's her story:

> *I went to the doctor and found out my son had thrush and I also had thrush on my nipples! It's not so noticeable in the baby's mouth because it's white, and your baby's tongue will look white from the milk. My doctor prescribed medication for my son and gave me iodine to put on my nipples. After a day or so the pain went away and it was completely healed.*

If you are unfamiliar with thrush, it's a fungal infection and easily spreads (think, if you have a yeast infection and you have sex, your partner will get it on his parts too). If you get pain after breastfeeding successfully for a while, get it checked and make sure you don't have an underlying problem like thrush.

You Have Enough Milk!

Don't stress about having enough milk. Stressing about not having enough milk will guarantee that you will not have enough milk. We all know stress will do crazy things to our bodies and one of those things is that it affects your hormones. If you are mentally stressed and keep telling yourself that you don't have enough milk, your body will deliver just that. The way to help your body produce more milk is to relax and have the baby on your breast. Milk production is a supply and demand situation. The more your baby demands, the more your body provides. This is one reason why not adding formula is so detrimental. At this early stage, it's even better to not pump milk and not use a bottle, unless you or your baby has medical reasons why he cannot be on the breast. A breast pump does stimulate the breast, but not the same way the baby does, and the more you have that artificial nipple in your baby's mouth, the less your nipple and milk production system are being stimulated by your baby and you are setting yourself up for possible problems later on. Also, it's much easier for baby to suck on that artificial nipple – it's like a beer bong. It just flows right in with little effort from the baby and he will not want to have to work so hard for his manna at your breast. Have confidence in your body's ability to provide your baby with what he needs. Don't focus on your baby's weight in the beginning and get all stressed out about your milk production. All babies drop weight after birth, in fact, they drop 7-10% of their birth weight in the first two to four days.

If you feed your baby and he still seems hungry, try emptying one breast before switching to the other. At the beginning of the feeding, your milk is waterier to quench your baby's thirst. The milk that comes in after that is hindmilk, which contains two to three times the fat as the milk at the beginning of a feeding. As you can imagine, this will be much more filling! The time it takes to get to hindmilk varies, it just depends on how efficient of a feeder your baby is. The takeaway here is, before you jump to conclusions and stress out that you don't have enough milk, try keeping him on the breast a bit longer to ensure he's getting hindmilk.

I want to advise you right now, do not even allow formula in the house at this early stage. If someone tries to bring it around, stop them in their tracks and send them back out. If you are worried about seeming rude, let someone else take it from the person and get rid of it through the back door immediately. Seriously, you don't need the temptation while you are working to get the hang of feeding your baby the way nature intended. You can prevent situations like this from happening if you are very clear about your intentions to give only breast milk from before the birth. It's not like you have to announce it to the world, just to those close to you who will be allowed to enter the house in the first two weeks – think: those who can see you in your underwear with your boobs hanging out (oh yes, and probably your in-laws, so you'll have to get dressed sometimes). Yes, you know who those people are in your life, and they will respect your decision!

OK, before you throw this book out the door, let me take it down a couple notches. My friends Peggy, Amy, and Michele all supplemented with formula a little in the beginning, for various reasons, whether it was that they thought that their milk didn't come in soon enough and their baby needed a bit more, that they couldn't get their baby to get a good latch in the beginning or that their baby was premature. The main takeaway here is that they were determined to give breast, so while they supplemented with a little formula in the beginning, they persisted with giving breast and were successful because they were determined to give their baby the best. So, it's OK, to give yourself a little flexibility if that's what it takes to calm yourself down and not throw in the towel because you just can't handle the stress. Just be sure you keep getting the baby to latch, offering breast first, before the bottle. Remember, it's supply and demand, so for your body to produce milk, you need to get your baby on the breast to demand it!

Augmented Breasts

A quick mention about those of you who augmented your breasts. I've known quite a few women with implants who breastfed their babies just fine, some for two years or more! The sheer act of getting a boob job doesn't mean you cannot give your baby milk, and research has shown that most of the time, women who think they don't have enough milk because they have implants is just perception, not the reality. The implant type (saline or silicone) and where it was inserted (in the nipple or under the breast) doesn't affect your milk supply. What MAY affect it is where the implant was placed. If it was placed behind your muscle, you should be good to go. If it was in front of your muscle, there's a slight chance you may have reduced milk production, but it doesn't mean you won't produce any milk at all. If you aren't sure about where your implant was placed, contact the plastic surgeon who performed the operation (if possible, and if not, another plastic surgeon) before you give birth to check you over and make sure you are all good. It would be very unlikely that you would not have any milk production at all, so worst-case scenario, you may have to supplement with formula, but always give as much breast as possible!

I want to share a story from my friend, Kathleen:

> *For some reason my daughter had a problem feeding off of one breast. I kept trying to feed her on that one side because I was afraid that feeding only on one side wouldn't be enough and I didn't want it to dry up. And you sort of feel like a failure to feed only on one side. Eventually, I realized that she was*

> *getting enough from the good side, so I stopped fighting it, let the troublesome side dry up, and was able to exclusively breastfeed her for 14 months from just one breast.*

Katherine didn't have augmented breasts, but she was able to exclusively breastfeed her daughter for 14 months on one breast. If she can do that, it should give you the confidence that you should surely be able to feed your baby with augmented breasts. Even if you have reduced production, you will likely still have enough to feed your baby, at least partially! If your baby really isn't gaining weight in the first week, definitely contact your doctor to determine what may be wrong. It may be your milk supply, or it could be something else entirely.

How Often Will My Baby Feed?

This goes back to moms worrying about their baby getting enough milk and also back to not stressing about it! All babies are different! Some will seem like they are permanently attached to your boob, 24/7, and with others, you may have to constantly wake them up to get them on the breast and keep waking them up during feedings. Generally, during the first week of life, most babies will gradually develop a pattern of feeding eight to twelve times in 24 hours. You should feed your baby whenever he shows signs of hunger – that means on-demand. I know some of you need a schedule: you have other kids at home, you have to work, you are anal and just need to know exactly when and how much your baby will be eating. If you are the latter, you need to let go a little, girlfriend. If this is your first baby, you will quickly figure out that babies don't behave according to plan. One of my best friends is this type. She had a really hard time in the beginning, adjusting to being flexible. We would take walks and she would be constantly looking at her watch for "feeding time." Her baby would not be able to sleep anywhere besides in her own bed, so she and her husband would always have to leave the fun early to get her home. In hindsight, she wishes she was more relaxed. So, use her experience as advice and chill out! Just let it flow and feed your baby on demand, especially in the beginning. Just plan to have your baby on the breast every few hours, including at night, and more often when she goes through growth spurts – and don't worry about it!

When you are breastfeeding, there's no way of knowing and you don't have to know exactly how many ounces your baby is getting. You can just tell if he's getting enough. Here are some indications to look for:

- He is gaining weight and growing as expected (this is the most important indicator).
- He has at least five wet, disposable diapers or six to eight wet, cloth diapers per day.
- She has two or more soft or runny bowel movements per day for around the first six weeks of life (babies have fewer bowel movements once they reach about six weeks).
- She is alert when awake, and reasonably contented.

If your baby doesn't have EXACTLY five wet diapers a day, don't freak out. The most important thing to look for is their growth – is she gaining weight as she should (within the percentile normal for her)? Of course, if your baby doesn't poop for days or there are no wet diapers, you should definitely contact your doctor. If something just isn't sitting right with your gut, contact your doctor. That's what he or she is there for, but use a little common sense, take a deep breath, and wait for a bit before you jump on the phone frantic that something is wrong with your baby, or worse, before you consider stopping breastfeeding because you don't have enough milk! You don't want me to come over there and thump you in the head, right?

Only Milk Needed

You DO NOT need to give your baby extra water or anything else when breastfeeding – breast milk is the most perfect, complete nutrition for your baby (except Vitamin D, but more about that in the nutrition section). I kept getting asked – don't you need to give the baby some water? I was even told, "When my babies were three months old, we would mix crackers in orange juice and give it to the baby." Yikes!!! Oranges and the juice are not to be introduced until 10-12 months or older, due to the possibility of causing diaper rash, anus burn, or even rash around the mouth of little babies. Imagine the effect of that acid on the immature digestive systems of such a tiny infant! Not to mention giving a tiny baby wheat products at such a young age! Yes, those babies survived, but

I imagine they had issues and the unknowing mom didn't know why. We know better now and have many opportunities to be educated about giving our babies the best nutrition we can.

Cracked Nipple Prevention

When I was pregnant and reading an ungodly number of books on everything to do with pregnancy and breastfeeding, a common theme was cracked, even bleeding, nipples. My friend Kim had a real problem with this:

> *In the first month, my nipples became dry and started cracking and bleeding. One time after feeding, my son threw up bloody milk. The nurse said it's ok, just pump on the bleeding side for two days. But after three days, my son threw up bloody milk again. My cousin told me she pumped exclusively for her babies, so I just decided to do the same thing.*

There's nothing wrong with exclusively pumping; at least your baby will get the benefits of drinking breast milk. However, you lose the convenience of just whipping out your breast and being ready to go, the bonding experience of having your baby on your breast, and some other benefits of baby suckling from the breast rather than a bottle. Cracked or sore nipples can be a sign that the baby isn't latching properly, so make sure you have a good latch. If your breasts are engorged, express some milk by gently massaging or pushing on your breast with your hand. You can also let warm water run over them in the shower to help release some milk. It's kind of like letting some air out of your tires so your car rides better, deflating them a bit may help your baby latch on easier.

If your latch isn't the problem, there are things you can do to prevent cracked nipples from happening in the first place. Try exposing them to the air after each feeding, allowing them to dry naturally. Avoid using soap on your nipples. Soap will wash away your breasts' natural lubricants. You can also rub some breast milk on your nipples – you'd be amazed at the healing powers of breast milk and what you can do with it. My friend Michele used breast milk and she swears by it! There are many products that you can put on your nipples to prevent cracking, like lanolin and coconut oil-based products, to prevent cracked nipples. I personally used lanolin and my nipples never cracked. I applied the product before I even had the problem, as prevention. You actually don't need to start using the product right away (like, don't pack it in your hospital bag). You can wait a few days to get the hang of things first. If you feel like you are having problems with baby latching on because of the slipperiness of the product, wipe it off before feeding or you can try using a different product.

If it's too late and you already have cracked nipples, there's research showing that putting a little aloe vera gel or a gel with 0.2% peppermint oil (if it doesn't affect your supply – see the section on herbs) works wonders – even better than lanolin or breast milk! Just be sure that you completely wipe these things off before feeding the baby, though.

Feeding Comfortably

Hopefully, you will be doing this breastfeeding thing for at least six months, maybe even a year, or more. You need to find a way to get comfortable and make it an enjoyable situation, not burdensome. Sounds impossible, but trust me, before you know it, you will be a pro!

Besides preventing cracked nipples, the most important thing you can do to ensure long-term success is to find ways to get comfortable, for both you and your baby. I already mentioned getting a comfortable rocker glider chair and a nursing pillow. This will actually allow you to multitask – feeding and catching up on things at the same time. However, I don't recommend sitting on your phone the whole-time baby is feeding – this is bonding time. Many times, your baby will fall asleep and it's just so comfy sitting in that rocking chair, staring at your beautiful baby laying in your lap. Enjoy those precious moments because, in a blink of an eye, they will be gone!

I'm sure you heard the advice – sleep when baby sleeps. This is most certainly true in the beginning. The best thing to do is when it's baby's time to take a nap, you should take a nap too. When I was trying to figure things out with my firstborn, I would prop myself up in bed on pillows and basically sit up in bed holding my son on the breast. I was completely exhausted, but I couldn't really relax this way. I knew I had to find a different position, so I started researching. The best one for me was to lay on my side with my baby lying in bed next to me, feeding on the lower breast closest to the bed. So, my arm closest to the bed would be up under my head or under the pillow, and the other arm wherever it was comfortable. I learned to do this on both sides. This position was invaluable to me because I could use it during the night too. I didn't have to worry about him rolling off the bed because the co-sleeper was there! My friend Peggy got relief from back pain using this position:

> *With my first, my back would hurt from sitting up. The weight of my breasts and the weight of the baby all on the front put a real strain on my back. It was so helpful when I learned to lay down and feed.*

When my baby would wake up at night (in the co-sleeper), I could just bring him in next to me, put him on the breast in this position, and doze a bit while feeding. I know what you are thinking – aren't you afraid to roll over on top of the baby when you fall asleep? I can tell you, your motherly instincts just don't naturally let this happen. You are asleep, but always a bit conscious. If this sounds weird, you will understand once you become a mother. You will never sleep the same way again! You just have to be smart about it, like if the baby and your partner are on the same side, put a pillow between you. If you are just unsure about falling asleep with your baby on your breast (like if you have exceptionally large breasts), then don't do it. And it should go without saying, never sleep with your baby in bed with you while under the influence!

Help in the First Weeks

If you are in a situation where you can hire a nurse to help you in the first weeks, do it! It doesn't have to be all day, every day, it can be just a few hours, a few times a week. The nurse will help you with any breastfeeding issues, helps with the first bath (and helps Daddy give the first bath too!), monitor the weight of the baby and other health checks, and just be there to answer questions. I loved having the nurse come to help and having her available to answer questions I had. When I had my second baby, I didn't really need her for the same things as I did the first time around, but what she did was help me with my older child: preparing food, giving him a bath, etc., which was a blessing when dealing with a newborn.

If hiring a nurse is not an option, you can ask a supportive friend or relative to come help, preferably someone who has had babies of her own and has some experience. You can also look up your local Women, Infants and Children (WIC) center. They have a great website with helpful resources, as well. Check the appendix for the reference.

You should also consider having a lactation consultant on standby, in case you need one. It would be good to find one ahead of time, rather than wait until you are desperate and frantically looking for one you sync with. A lactation consultant will give you individual, personalized help and she can do this online, so you don't particularly have to look for one in your neighborhood. My friend Anita would have greatly benefited from having the help of a lactation consultant:

> *I was very stressed when I tried to feed my baby. My breasts were huge, my nipples were also huge and bleeding, and I was staying with my mother-in-law at the time, who was not supportive of me breastfeeding at all. I didn't know which resources to turn to for help. My husband finally convinced me that I can still bond with my baby, even though I couldn't get her on my breast, so I exclusively pumped for six months.*

Thankfully, Anita was able to give her baby breast milk, but if she had help, she could have gotten through those challenging first weeks and been successful at getting her baby on the breast. She may have even provided her baby with breast milk for a longer period because feeding at the breast is so much easier than exclusively pumping.

Chapter 4
Oh, Those Visitors!

Now that you're at home, new baby in the house, guess what, everyone wants to come to see the new addition to the family! I will tell you right now that you need to stand strong and lay down some ground rules right away – and your significant other needs to be in on it with you. Believe me when I tell you that you will be in your pajamas all day, at least for the first few days. You will be getting the hang of the routine, getting the hang of breastfeeding, and getting to know the baby. You will have your boobs hanging out – even just being topless (if you are so inclined) since the baby will need to have access to your breasts most of the day. The last thing you need is to have to deal with people coming in the house and worse, asking you for things to eat and drink. Really choose who you want around you: Your mom? Your mother-in-law? Your sister? Your best friend? You need to only allow those who will be supportive. You don't need to have anyone around you who will make you doubt yourself with breastfeeding your baby. For family members who may be difficult to keep away, you need to be very clear about your intentions before the birth so they know what you will not find acceptable. It seems harsh, but one moment of hurting someone's feelings outweighs the benefits of providing the best for your baby in the long term.

One of the things I did to curtail the problem of visitors was post a sign over the doorbell at the front door; you can put it in a place most easily seen by visitors passing by. It had the baby's name, birth date, height, and weight – basically, all the things people want to know. Plus, it had a date and time when they could come over to visit – a baby viewing day. I set it for two weeks out from the birth date so I would have enough time to get settled and comfortable with the baby. Of course, you always have people who don't think it applies to them (I let my husband handle those people), but most people would drive up, read the sign and drive away. It really worked out perfectly and I did the same thing again when my daughter was born.

Mothers-In-Law

I have heard it all when it comes to mothers-in-law: doesn't support breastfeeding, makes you feel guilty for not breastfeeding, feeding too much, feeding too little, always around and interfering – it goes on and on. This is a very touchy subject because she's your husband's mother, so you can't just get rid of her (though you may want to!). You have to find a way to deal with it. My friend, Jane, really wanted to breastfeed her second baby because she was unsuccessful with the first. I went to help her and give her support. Jane was stressed, the baby was screaming, and the whole time her mother-in-law was sitting there next to her saying, "Poor baby." Not exactly the best scenario for success. Unfortunately, Jane didn't succeed in breastfeeding her baby because she just didn't have the support she needed.

First, you need to have your husband or significant other on your team; you need to have a unified front. You may not agree on everything, and in some cases, you may have to just let some things go, but you need to find the "don't cross the line" items that you will stand strong about. The biggest one may be that you want your baby to be exclusively fed breast milk. There's a generation of mothers-in-law who tend to be the formula generation, so they don't understand why you won't just give your baby formula. What I advise you to do first is be very clear about your decision to exclusively breastfeed BEFORE the baby is born. Hopefully, you will deal with this issue beforehand and not have to deal with it while you are learning the whole process yourself with a hungry, screaming baby. If she's not getting it, start showing her some literature about the benefits of breastfeeding and why you are choosing to do so. If that's not enough, take her to talk to your pediatrician or OB. If an authority figure like a doctor explains why breast is best, she may be convinced. Hopefully, these things work, but if she's a tough battle-ax, you may have to respectfully tell her that it's your decision and have your significant other with you to back you up. But definitely stand your ground and don't let her overpower you to the point where you compromise your principles!

Some women are in a situation where they need their mother-in-law, or even their own mother, watch the little ones when they return to work. This is where the real issues begin because she has the baby all to herself and you aren't around. Again, you need to pick your battles here. If she happens to put a diaper on backward or put on clothes that you don't like, this isn't a big deal, really. However, giving formula instead of breast milk, when you've explicitly told her you are exclusively breastfeeding, is off-limits. You may also have the issue of grandma (or any caregiver) overfeeding, causing baby to not want to nurse when he's with you because he's full, or underfeeding, and she's screaming from hunger when you pick her up. You need to choose what's important for you and stand your ground. For me, giving formula would be an absolute no-no and if she continues, I would find another sitter. Perhaps for you, it would be something else. Don't feel there's no way out – there's always a way. Don't accept something that totally goes against your beliefs because you feel stuck. You are never stuck, there's always a solution!

Part III
The One Year Stint

The American Pediatric Association recommends nothing but breast milk for the first six months of life and breastfeeding continued until at least one year. The World Health Organization recommends continuing breastfeeding for two years. In any case, you cannot give the baby regular cow, other animal, or other milk for the first year of life – it has to be formula or breast, so why not just give the best? My motto was, if the baby must have breast milk or formula, I will choose breast!

Chapter 5
Getting Out There

You have probably heard that you cannot take your baby out of the house until she is six weeks old. I don't know about you, but I got stir crazy after two weeks (really before that!). Of course, I wasn't taking my baby out in public at that time, but just going to my family's house was a treat!

The best thing about breast milk is that it's always ready, always at the right temperature, and always accessible. No need to worry about warming up the water or making sure the water is not too hot. I'm sure you've experienced it out in public – baby screaming, parents scrambling to get the water at the right temperature, digging in the diaper bag for the formula, trying to pour the powder in the bottle while juggling the baby, doing the mixing dance – all before hungry baby can get her milk! Yes, I know, they now have insulated bags to keep the water warm for formula feeders, but it's still just not the same as having it all ready to go. You still have to check the water temperature, mix the formula, etc. Take a look at women making formula when you are out – it looks like a Tik Tok dance! Pay attention next time. You will definitely think about me and try not to laugh! Many times, while out in public, I would discreetly put fussy baby on the breast with no one around me the wiser, and feel so glad that I was breastfeeding!

While you are with close family and friends with whom you feel comfortable, you may not worry about whipping out your boob when it's time to feed your baby. However, once you start going out in public, you may not be so comfortable with that, and maybe not the people sitting at the table next to you either. I know, it's a natural thing and it's beautiful, but we want to show the world that breastfeeding can be done discreetly, anywhere. We don't want to have to leave our enjoyable conversation to go to a separate room somewhere! So, showing some respect and discretion will go a long way in helping this cause. OK, yes, I've heard the argument that many non-lactating women wear tops where their breasts hang out in a very provocative way as a regular part of their wardrobe, so what's the problem with breastfeeding? I can agree with that statement, but my point is that we get much farther with sugar than vinegar, so why shove it in people's faces? This is my opinion, of course! If you want to whip your boob out in public and show people that you are going to openly feed your baby no matter what, then you go right ahead!

Some women are uncomfortable with the idea of breastfeeding in public, and many will just pump and give the pumped milk in a bottle when out in public. You can do this, but it takes away the convenience of breastfeeding. There are all kinds of things you can do to feed discretely in public and I think I tried just about all of them. First is investing in some nursing bras; you will need them whether you want to be discreet or not because they give easy access. These have been around for ages (I remember my stepmother wearing them when feeding my siblings when I was very young). What has become more mainstream in the past couple of decades is tops that have breast access. Yes, there are actually nursing tops. Some of them are God-awful, but some can be quite fashionable. Most of your favorite maternity stores will carry them, or all you have to do is search, "breastfeeding tops" or "nursing tops" online and you'll find an endless supply. In the first six months, when you are exclusively feeding your baby breast milk, these tops are a lifesaver. They have a discreet opening somewhere, so you don't have to lift your whole shirt up around your neck to give your baby access to your breast. If you are really uncomfortable with the idea of feeding in public, get one of these tops and try it at home first. Once you get the hang of it, you will find that no one will even notice you are feeding!

There is also a breastfeeding apron. Someone gave me one of these as a gift when I had my little girl, but honestly, it wasn't my favorite. It did give me some flexibility in what I could wear (it could be a strapless top, for example), but I found the thing hot and my daughter kept pulling it to the side like she was playing peekaboo. Perhaps it works fine if your baby is too small to pull the apron to the side, but it's also not very discreet, if you are worried about that. It's rather obvious what's going on when you hang a big apron around your neck. Not that you need to hide that you are breastfeeding, but it's just nice to continue what you are doing with no one being the wiser.

Baby carriers and other baby-wearing devices are more known for transporting your baby or "wearing" your baby, but they are also excellent as discreet breast-feeding devices while in public. I carried both of my babies in carriers for over a year – my son in a forward-facing carrier and my daughter in a sling. Not only did I love that it let me have my hands free, but I could do just about everything with them in there (well not EVERYTHING!), like cooking (not at the stove!), watering the plants, hiking, shopping, etc. How do you breastfeed with your baby a carrier, you ask? Well, in a forward-facing carrier, remember that your baby can face out, but can also face in. Normally, facing in is reserved for very wee ones, but the position can be used at any age. You just turn your baby around, lower the straps so that he is at breast level, and let him latch on. I walked all around Manhattan with my son like that. I even did a tour of a naval ship with him like that and no one was the wiser. This is when those discrete breastfeeding tops come in handy because no one can see your boob or that the baby is latched on. It just looks like baby is sleeping or chilling. Very sneaky and works like a charm!

When my son was around 13 months old, I discovered the sling and loved it because it helped support his heavy weight on my hip. When I had my daughter, I mostly used the sling, and I loved using the sling too. You don't have both hands completely free, like with the forward-facing carrier (which I still used for hikes and when I needed both hands free), but it's awesome for holding your baby close, at home or in public, and no one can see if she's feeding at the breast because her head is nestled in the sling. You can switch the sling to either shoulder, so you can nurse on both breasts. Admittedly, you do tend to favor the breast opposite your dominant hand so you have it free to use to eat, write, or whatever. For example, I'm right-handed, so my left breast got most of the action. You can easily balance it out by feeding primarily from the other breast when at home. I started taking a language course when my daughter was around 2 months old and I brought her along in the sling. When she started to fuss, I could just put her on the breast and she was quite content.

In the end, it's all up to you. Whatever you prefer, whatever is easier, more convenient, most comfortable for you is what's best. Use your gift registry to your advantage and let friends and family purchase these items for you.

Go to **www.heathermichellenutritionist.com/goodies** to see what I used for my babies.

Peer Pressure

While pregnant, you may make a friend group of other moms, like during pregnancy yoga, aqua aerobics, or birthing classes, and after your babies are born, it's very nice to hang out together and trade horror stories about how you aren't sleeping at night, baby pooped or peed all over you, or nice stories like the baby smiled, etc. Hopefully, most of these moms choose to breastfeed and you can help each other and trade stories about that too. However, you may encounter moms who did not choose to breastfeed or have other reasons why they aren't breastfeeding. In that case, you may be the only one whipping out your boob to feed your baby and you may start to feel self-conscious about it. This happened to me. I had a group of women who were all due around the same time as me, so we did stuff together, during pregnancy and after the babies were born. None of them chose to breastfeed and when I lifted my top to nurse, I would get these looks that made me feel uncomfortable, like I was an outcast. Maybe it was my own perception, maybe they themselves were feeling bad that they didn't breastfeed their babies, who knows? Since I was determined, I continued, regardless of the glances or insecurity I felt. My point is, do not EVER be embarrassed or intimidated! When no one else in your friend group is breastfeeding, have confidence that you are doing the best thing in the world for your baby. If you still aren't comfortable, perhaps you should consider finding a different mom group that has values more in sync with yours.

Talking about finding a mom group with values more in sync with yours, I'm not just talking about women who choose not to breastfeed, it can also go the other way. My sister was having trouble with her milk production when her son was around six months old, so she went to a group for support. When she got there, most of the children still feeding were not babies anymore, but toddlers, some even five years old. My sister was very uncomfortable with this and never went back to the group. My friend Randi had the same experience. Of course, we all have to do what works for us, and if that's your values, then that's the group for you! But it made my sister feel uncomfortable, and in the end, she didn't get the support she needed and gave up breastfeeding. I was proud of her for at least making it for six months, but she wasn't ready to stop and could have continued with the right support. So, don't give up! If one group doesn't match your values, search elsewhere. I listed some places where you can find support in the appendix.

Aren't Babies Supposed to Be Chunky?

Getting out there, people always have something to say, and one of them is commenting on the weight of your baby. This plays on the emotions and insecurities of many moms because so many of us worry that our babies are too skinny, or not gaining weight as he should. As I mentioned before, people love to throw out their unwanted opinion and love to tell you what's wrong with you, your children and what you're doing. Even some doctors can stress moms out and make ridiculous recommendations, like to just give formula, without really discussing options to continue breastfeeding. My friend Lanie had this happen with her third child:

> Between 3-6 months, my son wasn't eating well and his growth rate on the growth curve started shrinking. My doctor recommended I stop breastfeeding and put him on a special formula. This was a super rough experience because my son wanted to continue to breastfeed and I had to try to give him the bottle instead. My doctor didn't even give me the option of supplementing (giving both breast milk and formula). In hindsight, I should have researched it more or gotten a second opinion.

This also happened to my friend Amy, but in reverse. Her baby was really chubby, so her nurse told her to stop breastfeeding. At the time, she didn't know what to do, so she followed the nurse's advice. But talking about it now, it just doesn't make any sense. So, before you freak out that your baby is too skinny or too chubby according to someone's notion of what it should be, take a look at your baby and consider what's normal for him. Has your baby always been around the 10th percentile and been just fine and healthy? Then you shouldn't expect to walk into the doctor's office for a checkup and expect him to all of a sudden be at the 50th percentile. Take a look at your baby. Does she look like she's a healthy weight? I know this is a subjective measure, but are there bones and ribs sticking out everywhere? Sunken eyes? Or does your baby look like a normal baby? Is she having regular wet diapers and bowel movements? Is she eating frequently? Does she generally have a good mood and have alert hours in the day (hopefully not so much at night!)? If you are concerned, do visit your pediatrician to check it out, but if he or she gives you an opinion that doesn't sit right with your gut, or doesn't even want to discuss the option of supplementing, rather than completely stopping breastfeeding, look for a second opinion. Of course, you have to be reasonable – don't keep looking for an opinion until you find the one you want (don't be one of those people), but just get a couple of opinions before jumping to conclusions and being pushed into doing something you don't really want to do (like stopping breastfeeding).

Chapter 6
Other Stuff You Should Know

There are several things I think are important to mention, but they don't fit neatly into one category, so they are just other important stuff you should know.

Human Pacifier

I used to always think that I don't want to be a human pacifier. I read all kinds of baby books, with all sorts of different theories, philosophies, and recommendations. It was really driving me crazy. I knew what I felt was right, but was torn by what I thought I should do. One day, I called my girlfriend Suzanne, whose advice I respected, and told her of my dilemma. She told me, "Just go with your instincts." That was the best advice I ever got. From that point on, I went with my gut and allowed my babies to be on the breast on demand, and I'm glad I did. Remember, babies are comforted by sucking; that's why artificial pacifiers, which mimic the nipple, are so popular. Also, being on the breast isn't only about feeding, but also about creating a bond. If you don't mind being that comfort for your baby, by all means, go ahead, enjoy it, and don't feel guilty about it. If you don't really like it, then take your baby off the breast when she stops swallowing or when you know she is done feeding and use the pacifier or whatever works for you.

When Can I Start My Baby on the Bottle?

When I was doing all of my reading during my first pregnancy, the recommendation was to not give your baby an artificial nipple until he's at least a month old. The reasoning, as I mentioned earlier, is the artificial nipple is so much easier for babies that they won't want to do the work to get milk from the nipple. However, in hindsight, I have to disagree here. All babies are different and with some, it will be no problem for them to switch between the two nipples, but others just won't want that plastic or rubber nipple after being used to the real thing. My daughter is an example. She would never take an artificial nipple! This makes it very difficult to get away on occasion (which is much needed to keep your sanity). When I needed to do something for a couple of hours, my mother-in-law, who so graciously watched her for me, would have to feed her breast milk with a spoon because she just refused the bottle! That girl went straight from the breast to a cup when I stopped breastfeeding (at 17 months). No fake nipples for her! So, in hindsight, I would have made sure I had the breastfeeding down pat (usually after around two weeks) and then start introducing a bottle with breast milk, instead of waiting a month. This gives you a break and also gives Daddy a chance to bond at feeding time. Of course, this is my girlfriend-to-girlfriend opinion and all babies are different. One thing I do want to recommend, if you can at all help it, is for YOU to not give the bottle, at least until your baby is a lot older and very established on the breast. Your baby will identify you feeding with the breast and others with the bottle. You don't want her to identify you as feeding with a bottle.

Yikes, My Baby Doesn't Want the Breast Anymore!

So, you decide to go for it, you give your baby the bottle after you feel like you are well established with breastfeeding, or you had to supplement for whatever reason, and, horror of horrors, he doesn't want the breast anymore? I know this may seem like the end of your breastfeeding days, but don't fear, there are ways around this and, with a little perseverance, you will have him back on the breast in no time. Some things you can try are:

- Put something tasty on your nipple, like gas drops, or even just some breast milk.
- Try a nipple shield – it may fake him out to think he's getting a bottle.
- Try different positions or try holding him in different ways, like in a sling or other carrier.

Like I said, patience and perseverance are key! Sometimes, it may take a while, so hang in there. Always offer the breast first, but if that's just not working, there's another trick you can try. Give the bottle, then slowly slip out the bottle and when he roots again, stick in the breast. A bit of nipple confusion may be the charm! Just keep in mind that every small win counts, so even if you only get the baby to latch for a few seconds, it's a win. Just keep going, and most importantly, stay CALM! Getting stressed will just set you back.

Ouch! Does He Have Teeth Already?

One day, I was feeding my four-month-old and all of a sudden, I felt a sharp pain in my nipple. I was like, what the hell? What is that – it can't be teeth? He's only four months old! But I put my finger in his mouth, felt his gums, and sure enough, two little teeth poking through the gums! Let me tell you, even the smallest bite on your nipple HURTS! As they get older, they start getting more active and curious, and when the teeth start coming in, it gets worse. So, what do you do? Not breastfeeding isn't an option, so you have to find a way to make it work. Have no fear, girlfriend. I've been through it and there's a way to teach your baby not to bite. First, you do not want to give your baby the satisfaction of giving him a big reaction; it then becomes like a game to him, and you certainly don't want to do anything physical like hit or shake your baby (I know that sounds shocking, but I had to say it). The best thing to do, in my opinion, is when your baby bites, you just take him off the breast and say no, calmly, but sternly. Make eye contact so he knows you are serious. Give it 5 seconds or so and let him have the breast again. If he bites again, you do the same thing, but withhold the breast for a bit longer. By the third time, if he does it again, take him off the breast completely, sit him up, close your shirt and let him know you are serious. If he's going to bite, he's not going to get the breast. This will definitely get the message across because your baby is not going to like you taking the breast away! Don't think this will be a one-time thing and then you are done. It will take a few times (some babies more than others), but it works! I also need to add that you may get a whole temper tantrum out of this. You need to stand your ground and not give in – biting your nipple is non-negotiable, right? If you are in public, you just have to go outside and let him have his tantrum.

No, I Didn't Pee My Shirt

I have to admit, I was lucky that I never leaked and never sprayed. I never had to use those little leak guards in my bra and could walk around braless with a tank top and not have to worry at all. OK, don't hate me and throw out this book! I do know that there are plenty of women who aren't so fortunate. They leak through their shirts and spray across the room at the drop of a hat. If you are one of these ladies, be grateful you have so much milk!

My sister told me this story:

> *I was sitting in church and my son was in the daycare. All of a sudden, I felt the letdown and knew they would be calling me any minute because my son was hungry. The service ended before they brought him to me and when I stood up, I noticed the whole front of my shirt was soaking wet because I leaked everywhere!*

Don't worry about being embarrassed about these things. When you are a mom, there will be plenty of embarrassing things that happen to you when you have kids. They will pee on you, poop on you, barf on you – you name it. Things you never imagined dealing with happen when you are a parent. If something like this happens to you in public, all you can do is shrug and say, "I guess it's feeding time!".

There are things you can wear in your bra to help soak up the leaks. There are the old-fashioned disposable breast pads, the eco-friendlier reusable breast pads, and breast shells of various shapes and sized that catch the milk. On Dr. Sears' site, he states that breast shells push against your nipple when you're wearing them, so they can actually encourage leaking and overstimulate milk supply. Another issue with the breast shells is, what to do with the collected milk? Some sources state that you can "collect every precious drop." However, other sources state that you should never give this milk to your baby because of the potential to breed bacteria due to the uncertain temperature of the milk. I think we have to use a little common sense here. You shouldn't wear them around all day and you shouldn't use milk that you've been wearing in the shells for hours. If you put them on for a shorter period, using any milk collected in them should be fine. When in doubt, ask your lactation consultant or doctor.

Clogged Ducts and Mastitis

If you've read up on breastfeeding or chatted with girlfriends about it, you have probably heard of problems that can come along with it, like clogged ducts and mastitis. These things can happen, I won't lie to you. Many times, these happen when you aren't allowing the baby to fully drain the breast or when you skip a feeding (causing a buildup), but you may just be prone to them for whatever reason. The best thing to do with clogged ducts is to get the baby feeding on that breast as much as possible. It hurts like hell, like shards of glass being pulled through your milk ducts, but this is the best way to get the clogged milk to clear and pass through. You can try warm compresses to relax the area to help it pass, take a warm bath with Epsom salts, fill an old (but clean!) sock with rice and put it in the microwave to make a heat pack, as well as massage, and dangle feedings (leaning over the baby and "dangling" your breast as you feed).

My friend Kathleen had major problems with clogged ducts with all of her babies. Here's what she had to say:

> *In the first month with my babies, I had problems with blocked ducts that were very painful, so I would have to sit with hot washcloths on my breasts. My parents were with me and they would take turns heating water, soaking a washcloth, and putting it on my breast. Then I would become completely engorged, so to alleviate the engorgement, I would clean cabbage leaves, put them in the refrigerator to get them nice and cold, and put them on my breasts. You have to be really careful to not use them too much, though, because they can really dry you up. So, I would get blocked and engorged, using the hot washcloths on the top and sides of my breasts to clear the blocks and the cabbage leaves to alleviate some of the engorgement. After around a month or so, it got a lot easier. And when I would feel a clog coming on, I used the hot washcloths right away and I could manage it.*

The jury is out about cabbage leaves. Some sources say they have no effect on "drying you out" and others say when you're ready to wean, use cabbage leaves to help dry up your milk. You have to see how it works for you, but it would be wise to err on the side of caution. Take it slow and if you notice an unwanted reduction in milk supply after using them, leave them for your coleslaw or sauerkraut.

Many natural remedies purportedly help relieve and prevent clogs, but I'll just mention a few here. One is sunflower lecithin. Lecithin is naturally occurring in many foods, including animal products and whole grains, so it is safe. The idea is that it can increase the polyunsaturated fatty acid content of milk, making it less sticky and therefore, less prone to getting clogged. There's no true recommendation for how much you should take, but the Canadian Breastfeeding Foundation recommends 1200mg four times a day. However, this is something to consider as a preventive measure than an immediate cure, like if you have recurring clogs.

Another natural method is to use a poultice of fenugreek or parsley. Grind up the fenugreek seeds, add hot water to form a paste, wrap the paste in a soft cloth and drape the cloth around your breast as you nurse or pump. For parsley, just puree the herb and use it the same way as the fenugreek poultice. If you happen to be very sensitive to parsley and you think just the sheer act of having it near you is affecting your supply (see the section on herbs), don't use parsley, use the fenugreek instead.

The best way to clear ducts is to let your baby nurse on that side and let her drain the breast of milk. You may have to do this a few times to really clear it, but be confident that it will go away. Also, try the recommendations my friend Kathleen gave, hot compresses to loosen things up and cold cabbage leaves to relieve some engorgement (very carefully!).

Many women are embarrassed to admit this, but they let their husbands suck out the clog. This is very common, so don't think you are a weirdo for considering it! I never did it because I didn't think my husband would know how to suck properly to extract milk (there's a real technique to latching, after all!), but many women have said they did it with much success, so do what works for you!

Mastitis is taking a clog to another level. It's inflammation of the breast tissue that is sometimes caused by an infection. Symptoms are breast tenderness, warmth/hot spots, swelling, a lump, skin redness, a fever of 101° F or greater and generally feeling ill. If you have symptoms like a high fever, flu-like symptoms, or blood (not from cracked nipples) or pus in your milk, make an appointment to see your doctor because you may need medical treatment. If your doctor recommends antibiotics, be sure you emphasize that you are breastfeeding so he can prescribe something safe for lactation and the baby.

I'm Dying for a Glass of Wine

OK, so this is a personal subject. Some of you may be like, no way I'm touching any alcohol while pregnant or breastfeeding! Maybe you aren't much of a drinker anyway, so it doesn't affect you much at all. But, me? I really love a glass of good wine, or that ice-cold beer on a hot day, or a nice cocktail when I'm in that kind of mood. Are we terrible mothers for having a drink while breastfeeding? I say no! But of course, there's a responsible way to go about it.

If you do enjoy having a drink and are really craving one, go ahead and do it. If you don't, you won't last long breastfeeding your baby because you will constantly feel deprived. It's like dieting. When you are told you cannot have that piece of cake, that's when you want it the most! You may be able to resist for a while, but eventually, you will give in. My point here with drinking and breastfeeding is that I don't want you to feel guilty if you have a drink, and I believe that it's better to have a drink and breastfeed for a longer period than feel deprived and give your baby formula because you just couldn't keep up with all of the deprivations. It's not just about not having a drink, but there are so many other things that you give up for yourself when you have a wee one that it just may tip you over the edge.

If you are still shaking your head, don't take my word for it. The CDC says that moderate consumption (one drink per day) is not known to be harmful. Even if you have more than one drink per day, it's not an indication to stop breastfeeding because breast milk has a lot of protective qualities, so weighing the cost and benefits, it's better to breastfeed and drink than to not breastfeed at all.

As I said, there's a responsible way to do it. There's a time when your milk has the lowest, or highest, alcohol content. It typically takes around 30 minutes for your blood alcohol level, and therefore milk level, to peak at its highest, and two hours for that drink to metabolize out of your system. Having your baby on the breast while sucking down your cocktail sounds like something out of a Bad Moms movie, but crazy as it sounds, that's actually the time when your milk has the least amount of alcohol because it hasn't had time to reach your milk yet. Since alcohol is water soluble, like caffeine, it flows between your blood and milk, so while it gets in your milk, it also flows out as your body metabolizes it. This means that the worst time to breastfeed is 30-60 minutes after having a drink and the best time is before, during or two hours after having that drink.

How much alcohol gets in your milk anyway? Well, it's pretty much the same as what gets in your blood. The legal driving limit is 0.08% blood alcohol. If you think about having a drink that has 0.08% alcohol, you probably wouldn't have any effects at all. This may shock you, but plain ole orange juice can actually have as much at 0.73% alcohol! Bring this back to your baby drinking breast milk with 0.08% alcohol and any effects would be nearly null (if your baby is a preemie, a newborn or has medical issues, best to err on the side of caution and avoid alcohol during that time). Besides the weight gain from those extra calories and the hangover, the biggest problem with drinking too much and breastfeeding would probably be your impaired ability to take care of your baby. It would be a terrible thing if you tripped while holding your baby and she got injured. If you really feel the need to party it up, hire a sitter.

It's not rocket science, but when you know you will want to have a drink or two, having an action plan will just make you feel better. If you know you are going to want to enjoy a nice glass of wine with dinner, feed your baby beforehand. You have around two hours before you will need to feed again (this is when exclusively breastfeeding – you will have more time between feedings when your baby starts to eat solids). After around two hours, the glass of wine will be out of your system. Now, I did say a glass, maybe two, of wine, not a whole bottle! You need to leave the real partying for later when your baby is older, not feeding as much and you can plan ahead by pumping, but at least you can enjoy a couple of glasses while your baby is younger. A good rule of thumb is if you are able to drive, you are able to breastfeed. You should know how you should feel to be safe to drive. If you are at that point, then you are good to go!

Talking about pumping, there's a trick to that too. I'm sure you've heard of women who "pump and dump." A friend of mine called breast milk liquid gold and I totally agree with her! I just couldn't bring myself to dump, so I would plan it. If I knew I was going out and having some drinks, I would pump before the drinks started flowing. Then, you refrigerate or freeze the milk for later use (I would bring a small cooler with ice packs if I wasn't home) and enjoy your evening! When my son was around 10 months old, my husband and I were invited to a destination wedding where we had to leave him for two nights. I brought my double-sided, electric, breast pump with me, which was a blessing! I brought that pump to the reception and pumped right there in the bathroom stall before I started drinking. It was quite funny because my friend was in the bathroom with me to keep me company and that thing was so loud – it sounded like a cow milking machine! But, it was worth it. I had cold packs and a mini cooler in the pump bag, put the liquid gold in there, and had the best evening ever!

I will tell you that, realistically, your baby needs to be at least six months or older and eating solids before planning a night out, unless you are lucky enough or smart enough (I'm not sure which), to have pumped a big supply and have it on hand. However, when your baby is so small, a hangover the next morning would really suck! Once your baby is eating real food, the milk feedings get spread out longer, so you have more time in between and more versatility. Hang in there, mama, you will be enjoying cocktail hour again before you know it!

Breasts are for Feeding, not for Sex!

You passed the deluge of milk coming in, no more sore nipples and your breasts have settled into a beautiful size. Nice and full – better than a boob job! If you were already large-breasted, you may not be loving the new breasts and this may not apply to you, but bear with me here. These beautiful breasts have not gone unnoticed by your significant other, believe me. BUT, you are just in no mood to let him touch them! Not only are you exhausted from just being a new mom, you think of your breasts differently. They are now no longer sexual objects; their purpose is to provide nutrition for your baby. I'm mentioning this because you are not alone in feeling this way, it's perfectly normal. Your partner may be tired too, but men are always ready for sex! It's not only feeling a little violated when your husband gropes your boobs, your *punani* may not be feeling up to it either, especially if you had a natural birth. If you had a C-section, your *punani* may be fine, but perhaps you still have discomfort from the incision. You get six weeks, doctor's orders, to get a break and keep your partner away. But after that six weeks, you can't hold him off any longer and have to go for it. Maybe you are one of those lucky ladies who's also raring to go at this point, but you are far and few between. I can tell you that the first time is typically not enjoyable, particularly after a natural birth – it hurts, especially if you had stitches down there (and don't even look down there for at least a year because it's not pretty!). On top of it, you aren't exactly feeling sexy, with the extra baby weight, the incision right above your love triangle (after a C-section), and, if you had a natural birth, hopefully you didn't look down there like I told you not to! But I promise it won't last forever and things will be back to normal before long.

The point I'm trying to make here is that it's normal to feel like your boobs are off-limits to your partner during this time. However, sometimes you have to just deal with it because you just can't keep him off those luscious breasts forever, nor should you. The most important thing is communication – explain to your partner how you are feeling, and also remember, he has needs too.

OK, I know that some of you ladies may be saying, what the hell? I just went through pregnancy, birth, dealing with this breastfeeding thing, clogged ducts and sore, cracked nipples, while he sits there all comfortable. He can at least just keep his bazooka in his pants for a few months! I hear ya, but it's difficult to empathize when you have no idea what the other person is going through, and men are just a breed of their own. Plus, he may understand mentally, but emotionally it will wear on him. I'm very lucky that I have a husband who came right out and told me that he needs attention too. It's so easy to get caught up in your new bundle of joy. If your husband isn't much of a communicator, don't forget about him. He may be the nicest guy in the world, but no one likes to feel neglected and it will wear down that emotional bank account. It's hard to think about it now, but one day, the kids will be gone and it will just be you and your partner again. You don't want your last child to leave the house, you turn around to look at your significant other and wonder, who the hell is this person? Make sure you take time out to connect with each other!

Nine-Month Slump

This happened to me with both babies. The breastfeeding thing is going great, your baby is now eating food, so you don't have to breastfeed as often, you can have little snacks for them to keep them occupied, rather than your breast all the time, and can even get away for longer periods for some me time. Then, right around the nine-month point, you just get tired of it. Tired of having to always wear something where you can access your boobs, tired of not being able to have a drink when you want, tired of pumping milk, just tired of the whole thing in general. At this point, you feel like quitting. You already gave your baby breast milk for nine months, that's three months longer than the six-month mark, and you have not given your baby any (or minimal) formula up to this point. In only three more months, your baby can start eating everything and drinking regular milk anyway. You need a break, so why not just stop now?

As I mentioned earlier, my choice was, if I have to give breast milk or formula, I will always choose breast. Remember the ingredients in that formula? It's just nowhere near a substitution for breast milk and you want the best for your baby. What about you, you say? You have needs too, right? Yes, you do, but think about it. In the grand scheme of things, what are another three months in the span of you and your baby's life? It will go by in the blink of an eye.

I have a confession to make that may shock you. I met a girlfriend for a weekend in New York when my daughter was around 10 months old and I just couldn't pump enough milk for the whole time, so I left what milk I could manage to pump and… a can of formula! YES, I just said that!! If you really need a long break and just cannot pump enough milk, you can give a bottle or two of formula at this point (baby is already eating regular food anyway). If that will help you to stick through it, it won't hurt to give in on occasion when you really need it. The point is not to make it a habit. This means you will still have to pump when you're away because if you don't, your boobs will explode. Plus, you want to keep the production going, but at least you can get out, and you can even take a nice, deserved weekend with your significant other or friends.

I just want to mention that if you have to go back to work and just can't manage to give your baby exclusively breast milk at this point, this is ok! Just remember, some breast is better than none, so even if you are down to one or two feedings a day, hang in there! Your baby is still getting benefits from your milk!

To finalize, this slump will end as quickly as it came. Once you get past it, you won't think about it again and when that year mark comes around, you won't want to stop!

Chapter 7
Getting Back to Work

Many of us have to eventually get back to work. Some of you may never want to leave your baby and some may be just waiting for the day to get out of the house. If the latter is you, don't feel guilty! We all need some intellectual stimulation and sometimes; you can go a little crazy just being around the little ones for what feels like 24/7. Being a stay-at-home mom is HARD WORK! Don't let anyone tell you differently! You have probably seen those memes where you need different professionals with many different hats to fill the shoes of Mom. It's really true. You feel like you are getting pulled all over the place and with your sleep deprivation and post-pregnancy brain, you just feel completely scattered! It's no wonder that some women crave the scheduled routine that work brings.

It IS possible to work and breastfeed too. More challenging, yes, but possible. This is the time that you need to invest in a good electric pump where you can pump both sides at once, or even the portable pump that you can discreetly put in your bra. You also need to plan ahead. Knowing that you will be heading back to work, it's a good idea to start pumping and freezing milk in advance so you have a surplus for when you have to leave your baby with the sitter or daycare. It will be much less stressful than pumping each day for the next day.

Of course, you will have to pump at work to alleviate the pressure you will get in your breasts as your milk comes in (and to prevent embarrassing leaks, if you are a leaker). That means that you will need to be able to take breaks to pump. Most employers will understand that you need to have this time to pump, so just communicate with your boss. There are ways around this that can be agreeable to everyone, like spreading your lunch break over three breaks, etc. You should know how to talk to him or her to achieve the results you want (you know, like how you used to talk to your mom or dad when you wanted to convince them to let you go to the party of the year, or take a weekend trip with friends, or borrow the car – you get the idea). Be inventive and make it a win-win. It's probably wise to start this conversation before you go on maternity leave so you don't have to deal with it when you come back to work with baby brain. My friend Peggy had to go back to work after three months with both of her boys and, after the first time, learned what to ask for the second time around:

> *After the first baby, it was a challenge finding the time and support to pump at work, but it didn't stop me because I was convinced it was the right thing to do and there was no other option. I had no private area to pump, so many times I had to sit in the bathroom, it was the only thing I could do. With my second baby, I spoke to the boss before I gave birth and requested a space in the freezer to store my expressed milk. I also asked for a blind for the window in my office so I would have privacy when I had to pump.*

If your boss really isn't going for it, you do have rights as a lactating parent. It varies from state to state, so check your laws (I included a link in the appendix). If you maintain your productivity at work, you will show your boss that you can provide for your family and still perform at work (yes, we are Superwomen!!).

Maybe you work on your feet, like a hairstylist, or you are in the medical field running around seeing patients. The best time to start looking for gaps in your day where you can fit in a pump is when you are pregnant and still have time to think and plan. There's always a way to make things happen when you want them bad enough – there's always a solution if you are creative. There are even independent pumps that you can wear in your bra and are very discreet. (more about that later). Make it your priority and make it happen!

Ok, ok, so you are still telling me there is just NO WAY you can make this happen. With all the best intentions, life isn't perfect and you shouldn't beat yourself up about it. Stressing out about it will make things worse and reduce your milk supply. My friend Amber stressed out way too much:

> *When I started working again, it was very stressful. I stressed about going back to work, I stressed about not having time to pump at work and I stressed about not having enough milk in the freezer. I was so stressed that I wasn't eating, drinking, or sleeping enough.*

If you are so stressed that you aren't eating, drinking, and sleeping, what do you think will happen to your milk supply? The most important thing right now is to produce milk, so just relax and do the best you can. If your schedule just doesn't permit pumping when you need to pump, then pump when you can. If you don't stimulate your breasts at regular intervals, your body will produce less, that's just the way it works; it's a supply and demand system. So, just expect that you will produce less milk as you extract less often. If you can at least get your baby through six months exclusively on breast milk and no formula, that's awesome. If it's three months exclusively on breast milk, that's great too. The idea here is some is better than none, so if it's really not working out and you cannot pump enough to give exclusively breast milk, then give breast milk as much as you can. If you stop pumping at work, your body will stop producing during those hours, but if you get the baby on the breast at home, your body will adapt to the feedings demanded of it and provide what's needed. You can still feed your baby upon waking, before going to work, after work, and before bedtime. Then your baby will only need formula two to three times a day while you are at work. Even if you can get your baby on the breast just in the mornings and evenings, it's better than nothing at all. Forget the all or none philosophy; you can give some breast milk to your baby and she will still benefit!

Now I Really Feel Like a Cow!

Work or no work, if you want to have a life outside of having a baby attached to your breast all the time, you are going to need to pump. If you want to meet up with some friends for much-needed adult time or share some of the duties with your other half, you will need to have expressed milk available. Girlfriend, I have to tell you that pumping is a pain in the ass, ask just anyone who has done it. Maybe you are one of those lucky women who can pump and fill bottle after bottle with milk to share, but most of us barely get a few milliliters at a time, especially in the beginning. This is why I call it liquid gold. But, I can tell you that it does get easier!

I was lucky enough to be a stay-at-home mom, so I thought I didn't need to invest in a whole electric pump system. I only needed to be able to pump enough milk every now and then, right? I got one of those little hand pumps, you know, you put it on your breast and you squeeze the trigger with your hand. The first time I tried that thing, I think I literally got two drops out. As you can imagine, I freaked out! First, do I not have enough milk (yikes!)? Second, how the hell am I going to get any time for myself if I can't pump any milk to leave behind? After getting only two drops from pumping, I put my son on my breast and he just guzzled – I could see and hear him swallowing. So, I definitely had the milk! You have to know that babies are much more efficient at extracting milk than a pump, so don't freak out that you don't have milk if you can't pump it into a bottle.

My friend, Anne, felt she didn't have enough milk because she couldn't pump much:

> *Even though my daughter was gaining weight and always stayed in the 50th percentile, I felt like she wasn't getting enough because when I would pump, I would only get four ounces.*

With Anne's uncertainty, and having to return to work, she ended up stopping breastfeeding at four months, but as you can see, her baby was growing just fine and four ounces is a good amount! As with most breastfeeding issues women perceive they have, the problems are mostly related to their insecurities rather than the reality.

Pumping is a learned technique, and after a while, I was finally able to get a (small) bottle pumped with that thing. However, after a few months of squeezing that trigger, I got very frustrated (and probably carpal tunnel), so I bit the bullet and invested in a double-sided electric pump, which was the best I could get at the time. What a difference! A good breast pump is one of those things that I'm telling you to invest in; it's worth every penny. It may even be covered by your insurance (see link in the appendix). It will give you the freedom you need to stay in the breastfeeding game for the long haul. You will eventually need some "me" time to keep your sanity and being able to leave milk behind for the sitter is the ticket to do it!

When I was doing the pumping thing, I had to hold my pumps in place because I didn't have one of those "freedom bras." I would sit in bed, hold the pumps with my arms, and have my hands free to type on the computer or do whatever I wanted. However, there are so many different options out there, nowadays. You can even buy pumps that you just stick in your bra and walk around, some are completely leakproof! This may seem strange to you now, but believe me, after having a baby, you will be doing and experiencing things you never even thought possible! Some of these portable pumps work with an app and are quiet and discreet, so everyone around you doesn't have to know you are pumping. These types are perfect if you are working, especially if you have a job where you need to be on your feet. However, they are quite pricey, and some of them require you to purchase the milk bags that catch the milk, so what you choose just depends on your needs and your budget. Maybe your insurance will cover it, so it's something to look into, especially if this is your ticket for success to pump at work.

Many women are totally in love with a silicone "pump" that works off of suction, not a motor, and there are many women who are not. It doesn't really "suck," like a breast pump, it has suction due to the seal created between your boob and the flange, creating a vacuum. It is excellent for women who leak, particularly those who leak with a baby feeding from the opposite breast. Why let all that precious milk go to waste in a nursing pad, right? Basically, here's the down and dirty: if you leak a lot and easily pump lots of milk, you may love using a silicone pump. You don't have to worry about lugging around a breast pump, it has no sound that goes with it that makes you feel even more like a cow, and you don't have to deal with all those tubes and parts like you have with a breast pump. On the other hand, if it takes everything you've got to pump out two ounces and you aren't a "leaker," this may not be for you.

If you haven't had your baby yet and have never breastfed, wait and see how your body reacts before you run out and buy something. You will have time, don't worry. If you are just so tempted to buy something because your BFF swears by it, stick it on your baby registry. Then you didn't bite that bullet yourself and have nothing to lose – hehe! If you end up not using it, you can most likely sell it if it's still unopened.

If you are having a challenge getting milk from your breast and into the bottle, you may need to check the size of the flange you are using. I never even thought about this before writing this book, and I can't help but wonder if I knew to try different size flanges if it would have made a huge difference for me. There are websites where they tell you how to measure your nipples to find the right size. I included a link to one in the appendix. You can also ask your lactation consultant to help you with this.

If you have the right flange size and are still having issues with getting more than a couple of ounces of milk when you pump, there are some tricks you can use. One is to pump one breast while baby is feeding on the other one. When baby is feeding, your body is releasing prolactin and oxytocin to produce and stimulate the letdown of milk. Your body is already in "milking" mode, so you will have more success with pumping. Another tip that worked well for me was to pump first thing in the morning. Once your baby is only waking once or maybe twice in the night, you will have more hours overnight with no feedings, so your body will have generated a nice supply of milk. I would let my baby feed on one side and pump on the other and then after pumping, let baby finish off on the pumped breast. You would be surprised how much milk is still there!

You can also try this one. I saw this on Facebook and loved it:

> *So, I tell my husband that massage really increases my milk supply. I try to time it so when my husband rubs my shoulders, I switch the intensity on my pump so that more milk comes out. I don't use my slacker boob either. You gotta show that you're really getting milk while the massage is going on. Now, my husband really wants me to keep pumping (because I've wanted to give up a bunch of times already) and "helps" by giving me shoulder massages. He thinks it's so cool that his massages help so much. It is very, very cool if you ask me. -Jennifer Kay*

Storing Milk

Now that you have this liquid gold, you want to make sure you keep it pristine for your baby! It would be a horror, like, chime in the Psycho music, if you go through all the work to pump and it ends up spoiling. Here are the general guidelines I've found to make sure your breast milk remains good and safe for your baby:

- Most resources say breast milk can be stored for four hours at room temperature no warmer than 77°F (25°C). I've seen some that say six to eight. To err on the safe side, keep it to four hours, but if it happens to go to five, you don't have to throw it out. Just make sure the temperature in the room is cooler than 77°F and it should be fine.

- From three to five days in the back of the refrigerator at a temperature at or below 39°F (4°C). It's not a bad idea to keep a thermometer in your fridge to make sure it's maintaining the right temperature.

- Three to six months in the back of your freezer at a temperature at or below of 0°F (-18°C).

- Six to 12 months in a separate chest-type freezer at a temperature below -4°F (-20°C). You need to make sure your freezer is consistently holding this temperature before you attempt to give your baby milk that has been stored this long!

Can I Mix Milk?

You may be wondering, is it OK to mix freshly pumped milk with refrigerated or frozen milk, or fresh milk with fresh that was pumped earlier? It has to do with keeping your milk at a safe temperature to prevent bacterial growth. If you add freshly pumped milk (fresh out of the boob, warm milk) to frozen milk, you will decrease the temperature of the frozen milk to a point that could promote bacterial growth. The same with refrigerated milk – adding freshly pumped milk will lower the temperature of the milk into the danger zone. The way to combine milk is to get them as close to the same temperature as possible to prevent a big drop in temperature once they are combined. So, refrigerate your pumped milk before adding it to older, cold milk. You could even add refrigerated milk to frozen milk, just be sure it has been in the fridge for at least an hour before doing so.

You can mix fresh with fresh if you are pumping more than once within a four-hour window. Once your pumped milk reaches the four-hour mark (some sources say longer, but let's say four hours), it needs to go in the fridge anyway. Keep in mind too, that your milk is only as fresh as the oldest milk in the bottle. So, if you add freshly pumped milk to four-hour milk, the whole bottle becomes four hours old. Make sense? It's the same when adding fresh to refrigerated or frozen. The whole bag becomes as old as the oldest milk in the bag.

It goes without saying that fresh is best. Once it's stored for a while, it tends to lose some of those valuable antibodies and the composition of the milk does change over time. However, we do need to be able to get away sometimes, like back to work, or just a night out with our significant other or friends, and need to have milk available for other caregivers. Besides, correctly stored breast milk is better than formula any day! When using your stored milk, just remember FIFO – First in, first out. Use the oldest milk first. This means that you need to be sure to date your milk before you store it away. Keep in mind that thawed milk needs to be used within 24 hours. If you have leftover milk from a feeding, use it within an hour.

It should go without saying that you should NEVER microwave your breast milk! You can thaw frozen milk by thinking ahead and putting it in the refrigerator (I know, in a perfect world, right?), or putting it in warm water or a bottle warmer. If you don't have enough thawed frozen milk for one feeding and have some fresh milk available, give your baby the fresh milk first, then the thawed. Why the hassle? Because freshly expressed milk has all those awesome antibodies and other components that tend to subside when freezing milk, so you want to get that into your baby first, then the thawed. That way, if she doesn't finish the feeding, it's better to get rid of the older milk.

Talking about getting rid of milk, you don't actually have to toss it out. You can use it for rashes, cradle cap, cuts, and scrapes (for mom, dad and siblings too!), even in a bath! You'd be amazed at the healing properties of breast milk!

You want to be extra careful with pumping and storing milk if your baby is a preemie because he will be more vulnerable if the milk has any contamination. Be sure to be extra vigilant in sterilizing all equipment and keeping yourself very clean when pumping to avoid contamination. Fresh is always best, but breast milk, all or some, fresh or frozen, is better than none, so do what you can to provide your preemie your milk in a safe manner.

What Happened to My Milk?

There are many reasons your milk supply can seem to decrease. A big one, as I mentioned above, is due to stress. So relax, Mama! And before you freak out about losing your supply, there are many reasons why it may seem you are producing less milk, but maybe you really aren't. Before you throw in the towel and reach for that can of formula, seek some support or do some troubleshooting:

- Did you feed less than usual for the last couple of days for whatever reason (Remember, feeding stimulates milk supply more than anything else.)?
- Perhaps your baby is going through a growth spurt, so is on the breast all the time, in which case, has nothing to do with you producing less, he's just demanding more.
- Did your baby start sleeping through the night (One or two fewer feedings in 24 hours may cause less milk production.)?
- Are you having your period (This can cause your milk supply to go down.)?
- Did you eat a big bowl of tabbouleh (parsley can affect milk supply) or eat a peppermint candy or something else that may affect your supply (See the nutrition chapter.)?
- Have you been trying to lose weight and have restricted your food intake or started taking supplements for weight loss?
- Are you drinking enough fluids?
- Do you think your supply is down because you are pumping less than you did before?
    - Maybe your pump has been around for a while, so perhaps you can try changing the parts or the motor.
- Do you think your baby isn't gaining (but haven't weighed him) or someone told you he's too skinny?
    - Is your baby really looking thinner (and didn't go through a growth spurt) or has she always been at a lower percentile (and that's normal for her)?

Don't listen to others – they are always ready to hand out unwanted advice and they don't know jack. You know what's normal for your baby. My son was a "skinny" baby. Everyone would comment about it and say it was because I was exclusively breastfeeding. Now, my son is a HUGE teenager, much bigger than all his peers!

Also, there are too many women who are trying different fad diets during this time because they are so focused on losing weight. Some complain about their milk supply going down. Duh! Of course, if you restrict calories, and hence, nutrients, your milk supply will most likely go down! Making milk requires a lot of energy and nutrients. Your body will put everything you have into making milk, draining you of nutrients if it has to. Eventually, you will feel fatigued (even more than you already do), and your milk supply will eventually suffer.

What's a normal amount of milk you should be producing a day, anyway? Remember, your baby's stomach is tiny, that's why he's on your boob all the time – he can't handle much at once. A formula-fed newborn can only consume around 2-3 ounces at a feeding. We can't really tell how much a breastfed baby is consuming, but it definitely wouldn't be more than that (and probably less). Using this logic, why do you think you should be pumping a whole bottle every time? Remember, in the end, it's a function of supply and demand. If your baby is demanding, your body will supply. Get your baby latched on as much as possible. If you start supplementing with formula, that means that your baby is demanding less of you, which will just lead you down the wrong rabbit hole. You can also try power pumping (pump in between feedings) to stimulate more milk production if you just can't get your baby on the breast as often as you'd like (for example, if you are working). And before you throw in the towel after trying what you think is everything and the book, contact a lactation consultant. I've heard the cries of woe from so many women who stopped too soon and later wished they'd tried a little harder. Hang in there, and if all else fails, remember some breast milk is better than none, so give what you have first and then supplement the rest as the last resort.

I'm going to say it again, stress is the number one killer of milk production. Check your stress levels before you freak out that you aren't producing enough milk and relax. You may also need to take a look at your protein and fluid intake. Both of these are essential for milk production and you may be lacking in one of these areas. I have more detailed information about what you need in the nutrition chapter.

After troubleshooting other possible causes, there are some things you can add to your diet that may help get that milk flowing the way you want it to again:

Coconut water

There are many great reasons to drink coconut water, apart from boosting milk production. It's low calorie, packed with some vitamins and minerals, bookoo electrolytes, and it tastes great! I'm lucky enough to get fresh coconut water daily, but not everyone lives in an area where fresh coconuts are abundant, so drinking packaged coconut water is the only option. Admittedly, since the store-bought coconut water has to be pasteurized, the flavor is different from fresh, but drinking packaged coconut water is better than no coconut water at all!

Since we are talking about breastfeeding here, let's talk about the benefits to you, the lactating mama. First of all, who doesn't love something delicious, that is also low in calories (at around 50 calories a cup)? It's mostly water and full of electrolytes like potassium, magnesium, and sodium, so it's very hydrating (think Gatorade, but 1000 times better for you and without the sugar). If you've breastfed before, I'm sure you can relate when I say that when you first start feeding your baby, water becomes like an oasis in a desert – you can't get enough! The fluid and electrolytes that coconut water provides really help replenish your needs better than plain water. I'm not saying plain water isn't great, because it's the best, and water is what you should mostly be drinking, but sometimes, you need a bit more.

You know the age-old saying that once you feel thirsty, you are already dehydrated? Our body has a "water lag," so once thirst kicks in, you've already lost fluid and if it goes too long, you will become dehydrated. Dehydration, which can occur with as little as 2% loss of your body weight, can affect your mental and physical performance, so if you are experiencing brain fog and fatigue (what new mom isn't?), it could be just exhaustion from lack of sleep and all the other nuances of being a new mom, but it can also be from dehydration. One way or another, make sure you're consuming adequate water and other fluids. I personally started drinking coconut water instead of coffee in the afternoon for a pick me up a few years ago and it really works!

Before you go out there and grab a drink touted to boost milk production, look at the label. Most of them are made of water, sugar, a bunch of vitamins and minerals, and even coconut water. You should be taking a post-natal vitamin anyway, so you could really skip the other stuff and just drink the coconut water. If you don't have access to coconut water or just hate the taste of it once it has been pasteurized, you could go for one of these commercial drinks and see if it makes a difference. Just watch out for the sugar content – limit them to no more than one a day and find one that has stevia or other natural sweeteners, if possible.

There are other health benefits to drinking coconut water, eating coconut meat, and consuming the oil, but I started going off on a tangent and realized that this is supposed to be about breastfeeding, so let's stick to that. If you want to know more about it, check out my resource booklet at:
www.heathermichellenutritionist.com/resourcebooklet.

Oatmeal
Eating oatmeal is soothing, which can boost the hormone, oxytocin, the love and bonding hormone. Oxytocin also aids in the let-down of milk. It's rich in iron – low blood iron levels can result in a decreased milk supply. It's also high in beta-glucans, a soluble fiber that gives cooked oatmeal that gelatinous texture and one of the reasons why oatmeal is touted as being heart-healthy. Beta-glucans can lead to the release of prolactin, the primary hormone responsible for milk production.

If you don't like oats or can't eat them, other grains have similar properties, but they tend to fall short in one of the above areas. Barley has even higher beta-glucans than oats, but doesn't have the greatest iron levels. You can add some brewer's yeast, which is high in B-vitamins and helps with the absorption and metabolism of the iron it does provide. Teff and amaranth have a good amount of iron, but fall short in the beta-glucans arena. Eating any warm cereal is soothing, and as I've already said ad nauseam, many of our issues are related to stress! You can try different grains at different times and get all the same benefits. A vegan doesn't need to eat every meal with all amino acids balanced each time because eating different foods throughout the day will add up; this is the same idea. So, mix it up and try some different grains, I dare you!

Flaxseed
I've seen many women mention that they use flaxseed to boost their supply,

adding it to their oatmeal, smoothies, and lactation cookies. But does flax really boost supply? Some women swear by it and if you believe it helps, then, by all means, keep going! Flaxseed is a healthy addition to your diet and is regarded as safe for lactating mamas and their babies, so no harm done. While I cannot find any actual research or information that directly relates flaxseed consumption to a boost in milk production, there's anecdotal belief that the omega-3 fatty acids and phytoestrogens in flaxseed can help with milk production, so it's one of those things that just depends on your own experience.

Regardless of milk production, it packs quite a nutrient punch. Just one tablespoon provides almost two grams of protein, a slew of micronutrients, and fiber that keeps you regular and acts as a pre-biotic for your gut bacteria. It's also a good plant source of the omega-3 fatty acid, alpha-linolenic acid (ALA). The ALA converts to DHA and EPA, which are greatly beneficial to us moms (everyone, for that matter) and the ALA does get into breast milk, which will then get to your baby. So, while the jury is out regarding flaxseed boosting supply, it has other health benefits making it worthwhile to add to your diet.

Brewer's Yeast
I also see a lot about using brewer's yeast to boost milk production, so I thought to include it here. Again, there's not much real evidence to support that it helps you produce more milk, but it has been used for years by women swearing by its effectiveness. Brewer's yeast is probably most known for its B-vitamin content, but it also supplies a good source of protein, and micronutrients, like chromium, selenium, and phosphorus. The dosage for lactating is three tablespoons a day, which may be hard to choke down, so start with less and build up. You can also take tablets or capsules, but the amount of brewer's yeast in them varies, so be sure to read the label.

Brewer's yeast does have some red flags for certain people. If you have an allergy to yeast, diabetes (because it can lower blood sugar), inflammatory bowel disease like Crohn's disease, are taking medications for depression, are taking anti-fungal medications, have gout, or something else that you think you should talk to your doctor about first, then definitely make that appointment and get the all-clear before supplementing with brewer's yeast.

Part IV
Nutrition

Since I'm a dietitian, I thought to spend a little extra time talking about nutrition, weight, required nutrients, and the like. So many of us are confused with all of the conflicting information out there. Plus, we all want the quick, easy fix and I'm here to tell you that nothing in life comes free! Anything really good you have to work for, at least a little. I'm going to give you some simple advice on what and why.

Chapter 8
What Do I Need and How Much?

Your milk will provide everything the baby needs for proper development, besides Vitamin D. Of course, since you are providing your baby's only source of nutrition for the first six months, you'll want to make sure you are eating nutritiously to give her the best. If your own diet doesn't provide the proper nutrients, it will affect the quality of your milk, as well as affect your own health.

You've probably already heard that you need extra calories while breastfeeding (more about that later). Besides requiring extra calories, your nutrient needs go up, as well. Some of those nutrients include protein, vitamins A, C, D, E, and your B vitamins, including B12, as well as folate, potassium, zinc, selenium, manganese, iodine, chromium, and copper. If you stick to eating whole foods and stay away from processed foods and fast foods (hence, white flour, white sugar, and unhealthy fats), you should get all your nutrients. However, you still need to take a post-natal vitamin to make sure you are hitting all your targets. I recommend a post-natal that has the amount of vitamin D you need, so check out my recommendations at **www.heathermichellenutritionist.com/goodies**. Also, look in the appendix for links to recommended daily allowances and adequate intakes for lactating women for various vitamins and minerals.

To prevent this from becoming a nutrition textbook, I'll just stick to some key nutrients here:

Vitamin D

One important nutrient that you should really supplement is vitamin D because it's not found in adequate amounts in breast milk. Why is vitamin D necessary, you ask? I'm sure you've heard about all of the benefits of having adequate vitamin D – it's like it's some kind of miracle vitamin. It's almost a cure-all for everything! It seems like every week, I see research showing a new health benefit of Vitamin D. In the case of your baby, the main thing vitamin D does is prevent rickets. You know, where bones don't get strong enough and a child ends up with bowed legs. There is also evidence that vitamin D deficiency during pregnancy can cause negative health outcomes, such as postpartum depression. More recently, a study found that pregnant women taking 4,000 IU per day of vitamin D had the greatest benefits. So, make sure you are getting your daily dose of D!

There is a great study in the journal, Pediatrics, with 334 mother/baby participants in two different geographical locations and diverse ethnic groups. The current guidelines are for babies to be given a supplement of 400 IU of Vitamin D per day. In the study, they gave mothers a range of doses: 400 IU, 2400 IU, and 6400 IU. The moms getting 400 IU also had to give their babies 400 IU. After a period, the moms getting 2400 IU were discontinued because the babies were deficient in vitamin D. The babies whose moms took 6400 IU had blood levels of vitamin D equal to that of the babies who were getting 400 IU supplemented. This means that at higher doses, supplemented vitamin D will pass into mother's milk in enough quantities to provide the baby with what he needs.

I know, 6400 IU sounds like a lot and vitamin D is a fat-soluble vitamin, so you won't just pee out the excess like you do with water-soluble vitamins, like vitamin C. In the same study, they addressed this issue. Within the past 10 years, the Institute of Medicine increased the upper limit to 4000 IU per day and the Endocrinology Society set the upper limit at 10,000 IU per day. If you know anything about upper limits in nutrition, there's always a buffer, so consider it a "play it safe" dosage. This means that you can feel quite confident that you will be safe taking as much as 6400 IU of vitamin D per day.

Omega-3s

Another nutrient you may have been told you should supplement is omega 3. The amount of omega-3 fatty acids in breast milk is directly related to your intake, so the amount you consume is directly related to how much is available in your milk for your baby.

Do you remember the old TV shows and movies where they showed kids being fed a spoon full of cod liver oil – yuck! Cod liver oil is full of omega-3 fatty acids. I have to admit, I did take cod liver oil while I was breastfeeding and it was nasty! There are all kinds of fish oil supplements available, so you don't have to do this. Plus, you may be able to get what you need by consuming fish weekly.

It was a bit overwhelming researching this topic because there's so much information, and then there's insufficient information, specifically on omega-3s and lactation. I'm going to keep it simple so it doesn't get boring and just give you the Cliff's Notes of what you need to know. There are two commonly known omega-3 fatty acids: DHA and EPA. I'm sure you've heard of them. DHA is critical for your developing baby's nervous system, particularly during times when brain growth is at its peak, which is late pregnancy and early infancy. DHA is also important for the development of the retina, particularly before birth, so it's important to consume adequate omega-3s while pregnant, as well.

What we do know is that DHA is critical for proper neuro and retinal development and that the amount in your milk is directly related to your intake. However, what we don't know is how much a lactating woman should be getting daily. I've looked at numerous studies and there's just not a clear-cut conclusion. One study in the Journal of Pediatric Gastroenterology and Nutrition was looking into this very topic, but was only able to come up with a recommendation based on what should be consumed to balance the loss of DHA in milk, which is 100mg a day. However, this is an amount just to replace losses, which may not be adequate for optimal health.

The American Academy of Pediatrics recommends 200-300mg of DHA per day for everyone. This can be taken in supplement form or consumed as part of your diet. According to the 2015-2020 Dietary Guidelines for Americans, pregnant or breastfeeding women consuming 8-12 ounces of seafood a week, choosing varieties that have the highest DHA and EPA profile and the lowest levels of methyl mercury, will help you reach that goal. You probably already know which fish are highest in mercury because you've been avoiding them throughout your pregnancy. The fish you want to eat to get the most amount of DHA and the least amount of mercury are salmon, sardines, herring, and trout. You may like salmon and trout, but are turning your nose up to sardines and herring. But, just give it a try! I don't have much experience with herring, but canned sardines on crackers are actually quite delicious! If you eat sardines with the bones, you are getting a great source of calcium too!

There have been no upper limits established for omega 3s, however, the FDA has stated that up to 3000mg per day of DHA and EPA is "generally regarded as safe." However, if you are taking blood-thinning medications, please consult your doctor before taking any omega 3 supplements.

I think the takeaway here is to consume your omega-3 in real food as much as possible and supplement the rest. I always recommend getting your nutrients from food first, because there are so many components in real food that we don't even know about that all work together for the best overall health outcome. So, eating the recommended 8-12 ounces of fish per week, plus a supplement containing at least 200mg should ensure that you are getting what you and your baby need for optimal health. If you are vegetarian or vegan, look for supplements from algae. Check out my recommendations for supplements at: **www.heathermichellenutritionist.com/goodies**.

Calcium

Calcium is one of those minerals that we have been told time and again that we must consume in adequate amounts for optimal health, namely to prevent osteoporosis. They tend to come in those horse pills and, I don't know about you, but I hate swallowing pills in general, so I nearly choke on those things! Lactation (and pregnancy, for that matter) is a period of high calcium requirement. This doesn't mean you need to take two horse pills, it means that your body uses more calcium than usual. Amazingly, your body adapts to these needs, regardless of maternal intake, so your growing baby and your milk are not affected by how much you consume. I know you are thinking; don't I need more calcium to replace what my body takes from my bone? That is completely logical, but there are actually firm data that demonstrates low calcium intake doesn't lead to exaggerated bone loss. I know some of you may be completely shocked that I'm saying this, but I'm telling you, study after study that I read all reported that there's just not enough evidence out there, as of now, to recommend lactating women increase their calcium intake. I did see one study that looked at a group of women in The Gambia where their calcium intakes were already low before pregnancy and lactation. The researchers concluded that their baseline low intake would be suboptimal for lactation, but if you are already consuming an adequate amount of calcium, you should be good.

With all that said, let's weed out the noise and come to a concrete recommendation based on what we know right now. Make sure you are always getting your recommended daily allowance (RDA) for calcium, (regardless of whether you are pregnant or lactating) to make sure you are at optimal levels when you do need the calcium for abnormal physiological processes, like lactation. The RDA for adults 19-50 years old (child-bearing years) is 1000mg per day. As long as you are getting that, you should be good. If you have a specific health issue where you need either more or less calcium, the recommendation may be different for you and you need to talk to your doctor.

Protein

As a lactating mama, you need to increase your protein intake by 20g per day while your baby is relying solely on you for her food intake. Needs are directly related to how much milk you are producing, so as the baby starts eating solids and consuming less milk, the extra protein needs go down to around 15g per day. What does that even mean? Well, an average person needs around 0.8 to 1.0g/kg of protein per day. If you aren't used to working with kilograms, multiply by 2.2 to get pounds. So, a 60 kg person (which is around 132lbs) needs around 60 grams of protein per day. Add 20g and you need 80 grams of protein a day. To put this in perspective, an egg has around 6.5 grams, a handful of almonds has 9 grams and a chicken breast has around 30 grams of protein. You may be thinking, "I probably get triple the protein I need with how much I'm eating!" Maybe you do, but moms with little ones tend to grab what they can quickly shove in their mouths and not really sit down to a full meal. If you are struggling with supply issues, a reason may be that you aren't getting enough protein. Just take a look at what you're eating and make sure you are getting at least three actual meals a day. If you find you are mostly snacking on crackers and the like, you may need to up your protein intake. Adding some protein with every meal and snack will help you meet your quota. In my resource booklet, I list the protein content of some foods at **www.heathermichellenutritionist.com/resourcebooklet**.

Fluids

Breast milk is mostly water (around 87%), which is why an exclusively breastfed infant does not need supplemented water, no matter what Aunt Edna tells you. This also means that your body will be using a lot of water to produce milk. This equates to a need for more fluid and believe me, your body will tell you – you will be parched like you've been walking in a desert for days! That's the old oxytocin at work – it makes sure you are thirsty so you get enough fluids. I can remember waking up in the middle of the night feeling so parched, I would just guzzle down a bottle of water that became a staple by my bedside.

According to the National Nutrition Survey in Australia, women in general need around eight to nine, 8oz (237ml) cups of fluids a day, including water, tea, milk, etc. Even though sugary and caffeinated drinks are fluids, in my book, they don't count and you should know very well why! If you aren't sure, shoot me an email and I'd be happy to stand on my soapbox and tell you!

The average milk production in the first six months is around 0.78 liters a day, which comes out to around 0.70 liters (around 3 – 8oz cups) of fluid. That means you need to replenish that lost fluid, so go ahead and add another half-liter or so to your normal requirements. There are adequate intake recommendations for fluids, however, fluid needs vary depending on your activity level, your climate, how much you sweat, etc., so there's no one-size-fits-all recommendation. Let's go with the Australian recommendation so we have a baseline. Non-lactating women need around eight to nine cups a day, add the extra half-liter and you are talking about around 10-11 cups of fluids per day while lactating.

The easiest thing to do to make sure you are getting your recommended daily

fluid intake is to have a container of a certain size, calculate how many of those you need per day to meet your requirements, and don't let it leave your side all day (wear it around your neck if you have to) until you've drunk all your fluids! For example, if you need 10 cups a day, that's 80 ounces (2.4L), so if you have a 26oz container, you will need to drink at least three of them to get near your requirements (remember, you get fluids from other beverages too). I highly recommend getting a stainless steel, vacuum container, or at least BPA-free plastic one, that will keep your drinks cold and not leach nasty chemicals in your water. You don't want to be working so hard to keep yourself and your milk healthy just to consume a bunch of chemicals. See what I use at:
www.heathermichellenutritionist.com/goodies.

A good way to make sure you are properly hydrated is to look at your pee. If it's yellow, you need to drink more. The darker the yellow, the more dehydrated you are. The paler the yellow, the better. It doesn't have to be totally clear, but at least a pale yellow, and if it's particularly smelly, you either ate a bunch of asparagus, or you need more fluids.

Get into the habit of always having a bottle of water around. It doesn't have to be rocket science, just drink up, make sure your pee is pleasant (as it can be) and you will be fine! And seriously, if you have a low supply, this may be the monkey on your back. Even if you don't have a low supply, just do it anyway. You need adequate fluids, regardless!

Chapter 9
Giving Up Your Favorite Foods – is it Necessary?

You will hear advice from all kinds of people about what you should and shouldn't be eating – both during your pregnancy and while breastfeeding. I remember being told that I cannot eat spicy food while pregnant because the baby won't come out clean! You will hear some crazy stuff, but also some good stuff from health professionals, and even girlfriends, which may help you. In the end, it's personal. What affects some women and babies doesn't affect others. If you have ever been around a crying baby who can't be soothed for anything, think about what you recently ate and try to avoid it for a while. But it's not all black and white, so it will just be trial and error.

There's a great study where they investigated food restriction during breastfeeding compared to the literature on the validity of these dietary restrictions and it appears that many women are restricting their diets unnecessarily. Common restricted foods include caffeine, spicy foods, gassy foods, raw foods, and cold foods. Did you just freak out when I said caffeine? So many of us are dependent on that morning coffee (which really isn't a good thing anyway – but that's another topic), especially after not sleeping all night with a baby in the house. Well, rest assured, it is OK to have and enjoy your coffee! The amount of caffeine transferred to breast milk is generally less than 1% of that consumed. No caffeine has been detected in an infant's urine with consumption of up to three cups of coffee per day. Once it starts getting up to five cups in a day, caffeine could begin accumulating in an infant's system, but how many people really drink that much (are you looking the other way?)? The recommendation for caffeine intake during pregnancy is no more than 300mg (around two cups of coffee), so just stick to that while breastfeeding and you should be fine.

Regarding spicy or gassy foods, they do not negatively affect breast milk. Spicy foods can change the flavor of milk, but believe it or not, it seems babies like a variety of flavors in breast milk, which can even help them prepare for the different flavors they will encounter when weaning to solid foods. One study found that infants of mothers who consumed garlic extract actually fed for a longer time at each feeding. Gassy foods may affect mama's bowel, but they don't pass into breast milk and neither does acid from acidic foods, so enjoy your sauerkraut, kimchi, and pineapple smoothies without worry!

The concern with raw foods, like sushi, tartare or unpasteurized milk, is food poisoning. However, this does not affect your milk, and will therefore not affect your baby. Food poisoning will affect YOU though, and it would really suck to be hanging over the toilet with a baby needing to feed, have her diaper change, screaming his head off, etc. So just be smart here and be food-safe, like you usually are. If you normally enjoy sushi, eat it! Just don't try the roadside sushi stand for the first time; go where you know it's clean and safe.

Talking about fish, excessive amounts of mercury can pass through breast milk and may be harmful to your baby. So, just use the same guidelines as pregnancy – avoid certain large fish: swordfish, king mackerel, and such, that are known to have high levels of mercury. The benefits of the essential fatty acids, like DHA, you receive from eating fish and seafood outweigh the risk of possible mercury overdosing, so don't avoid it altogether!

Some women don't consume cow's milk because they are afraid their baby may have a cow's milk protein allergy. Keep in mind that it's the protein that causes allergies, not the lactose (milk sugar). Research has shown that reactions to cow's milk proteins, in the amounts received in breast milk, are rare. It's actually babies fed formula, even when given formula and breast, who have shown some adverse reactions to cow's milk proteins. However, some babies just seem to be sensitive to dairy. This was the case with my friends Lilian and Lanie:

Lilian:

> *Neither of my babies liked when I ate dairy; they would get a rash on their cheeks. Soft cheese was a problem, older cheeses, not so much. They are still sensitive to dairy to this day. Asians generally tend to be sensitive to dairy, so this is probably why.*

Lanie:

> *I ate very simple foods in the beginning with all of my babies. I had to modify my diet or they would get gassy. Dairy was a big one that I had to avoid.*

Again, it's really individual and you have to see what works, or doesn't work, for your baby. However, it's important that you consume sufficient calcium, whether that be in cow milk, cheese products, or other sources. If you are concerned, you can always try goat's milk – I have a whole discussion about it later on, but it does not cause the same allergy issues as cow milk and is much more digestible. While the calcium content in plant sources tends not to be as bioavailable as animal sources, you can still meet your calcium needs without consuming dairy at all. Check out the resource booklet at: **www.heathermichellenutritionist.com/resourcebooklet** for a list of the calcium content of some foods.

If you find that there's a food that seems to cause a reaction in your little one, it is not necessary to avoid these foods the entire time you are breastfeeding. It's mostly in the first couple of months when your baby's digestive system is vulnerable. For my son, it was chocolate, and I learned the hard way. My son was born in January, and on Valentine's day, I indulged in a delicious chocolate fondue, and when I say indulged, I must have eaten a quarter of the whole fondue! A few hours later, my poor little boy was screaming and there was nothing I could do to get him to stop. Of course, I went hog wild with that chocolate and that's just not normal. Having a normal amount of chocolate would have been just fine.

Just remember that Mother Nature is programmed to protect your baby, so it will keep the worst components out of your milk. It will also pull needed nutrients into the milk, even at mama's expense, if you aren't consuming enough for you and your baby to get what's needed. Your body will warm your milk to the perfect temperature (yes, even if you drink ice water) and make sure it has the nutrients your baby needs (except for the vitamin D you need to supplement). Be confident in your body's ability to produce what and how much your baby needs for optimal growth!

The final word on this is that there are no foods that you absolutely cannot eat while breastfeeding. Babies will have gas no matter what you do, so don't stress out that your baby has gas just because of something you ate. Just be aware of your baby crying differently than normal (louder, clenched fists, pulling her legs into her chest) and then go back and think about what you ate and avoid it for a while or eat it in smaller amounts. If you have time, you could keep a food diary so it's easy to associate foods with your baby's behavior. If you see unusual reactions in your baby, eczema or other unusual skin reactions, excessive mucus, etc., definitely talk to your doctor to rule out any real food allergies or other causes.

Caffeine

OK, I just want to make a quick mention about caffeine. I know it's a lifesaver for many of you who are sleep-deprived, walking around like zombies all day. Without that caffeine fix, you just won't make it, right?

Well, I'm sure you know this, but I'm going to say it anyway. Caffeine is a drug and just like all drugs, caffeine has an adaptive factor. The more you consume, the more your body needs to get the same effect. What you might not know is the mechanism of how it works. You have a neurotransmitter, or a chemical messenger, called adenosine that's released to signal your brain that it's time to go to sleep, making you relaxed and sleepy. Caffeine actually fits on the same receptors as adenosine, but rather than make you feel relaxed and sleepy, it makes you feel awake and energetic. When you have a bunch of caffeine floating around, it takes up all the adenosine receptors, so it blocks the effects from adenosine. But, you say, what's the problem? This is exactly what you want, right? To block the tired feeling and get energized! The problem is that the effect is short-term. First of all, when the caffeine wears off, you have all this extra adenosine floating around that floods those receptors and makes you feel like you want to fall flat on your face. Then, your body isn't stupid. It knows that you are overstimulated and wants to get that adenosine in there to make you rest, so it produces more adenosine receptors and more adenosine. Now, you have to drink more caffeine to fill those extra receptors and it just becomes a vicious cycle. You need to drink more and more caffeine to keep filling up those extra adenosine receptors your body is making. Eventually, you end up feeling below-normal energy and clarity than baseline because your body is starting with less than zero. At this point, you need that coffee to just get back to baseline again (you know, you need that cup of coffee in the morning before your brain starts to function).

It's a vicious cycle and the only way to kick it is by detoxing. I know, I know, this isn't the best time to do this. I have to be honest and say that the detox makes you feel like crap - brain fog, fatigue, and it takes a good week or two, depending on how much caffeine you have been consuming a day, to start feeling normal again. So, I understand if now isn't the best time to do this. But what you can do is stop upping your caffeine intake. Stick to a certain amount per day – like two cups of coffee or equivalent (around 300mg). Then, if you need another boost, try something else. Move around a bit, stand up and stretch, put on your favorite songs and sing or dance. Exercise and movement always give an energy boost (and you may even get a giggle out of your baby watching you do this!). Go out for a walk, the movement will perk you up. Other ideas: Watch or listen to something so funny it makes your belly hurt; put some peppermint-scented oil on your temples, in an infuser or drink a cup of peppermint tea (if it doesn't affect your supply); take a cold shower; do the *Breath of Fire* (see my resource booklet at **www.heathermichellenutritionist.com/resourcebooklet**). I personally love to drink coconut water for a bit of energy. Whatever floats your boat is fine, as long as it's not loaded with added sugar and caffeine!

Chapter 10
Herbs – What Should You Know?

First of all, I just want to mention that I'm not a doctor, pharmacist, herbalist or holistic practitioner. I'm a registered dietitian, which means that I'm a nutrition professional who has limited medical knowledge, so I can discern if a research study or other information seems to have valid results or not, but I don't know all of the ins and outs of the effects of what every herb, pill or supplement may have in your particular case, so please consult your health professional who knows you, your health history, any medications you may be taking, etc. before trying something and then pointing your finger at me and saying that I told you to take it!

Second, herbs aren't as thoroughly researched as we may like because, well, research costs a lot of money and you can't really charge much for herbs that people can literally just grow in their yard (mostly). So, while there are some studies out there, many of them aren't really conclusive.

Keeping that in mind, some herbs are rumored as being helpful, or detrimental, to milk production. Like with almost everything, we are all unique individuals and what may work for one person may not work for you, so you will have to do a bit of trial and error and fine-tune what works best for your milk supply. The most important thing is making sure you are doing trial and error with things that are generally safe. This isn't an exhaustive list, in fact, I will just touch on a few herbs that are widely discussed in relation to lactation, but in the appendix,

I include some sites that have, what I believe to be, research-backed advice.

Herbs That May Boost Supply

Fenugreek

Fenugreek is touted as one of the best lactation stimulating herbs and has been used for this purpose for centuries. What is consumed is the seeds of the fenugreek plant. The seeds have fiber, protein, iron, magnesium, and manganese, all good for you lactating mamas. There have been some studies showing positive effects of fenugreek on milk production. In one of the studies, the infants regained their birthweight faster than those whose mothers didn't take the herb. Most of the studies did not use fenugreek alone, but in combination with other herbs, nutrients, etc., as a tea or in a supplement form, so it's unclear if it's the fenugreek or the combination with other things. However, the one common denominator in all the products studied was fenugreek, which is a mark in favor for this herb in particular. It was reported that you need to take it consistently to get results. If you take it now and then, you may not get the boost in supply you are looking for. You have to be patient as it can take anywhere from 24-72 hours, and even as long as two weeks, to see results.

There have been some side effects reported in nursing mothers taking this herb, but it's difficult to determine if it's from the fenugreek itself, or something else. They include gassiness, stomach upset, and diarrhea – even mom and baby smelling like maple syrup, which doesn't seem so horrible! The most common complaint is gassiness in the mother and baby. You can try fenugreek in a supplement, tea, powder or even snack bars and see how it works for you. Take note that this herb is also known to lower blood sugar levels, so if you have issues with your blood sugar, please consult your doctor before trying this out. Also, if you are allergic to chickpeas or peanuts, have asthma, or have a history of estrogen-receptive cancer, consult your doctor before taking this herb.

There's a lot of information about fenugreek, so please look at the appendix for sites and articles on the subject with more information. There's a product line that I like that has fenugreek and other herbs and nutrients that can help boost your supply! Check it out at **www.heathermichellenutritionist.com/goodies**.

Fennel

When my son was a baby, and I was dealing with the dreaded colic, I was told about fennel, as in the fennel seeds. I would make some fennel tea and give him a little by the spoonful (cooled, of course!). What I didn't know at the time was that I should have also been drinking it myself. Fennel is known to stimulate breast milk production, but is particularly known to relieve gassiness and stomach upset (hence, giving it to a colicky baby). If you get stomach troubles from fenugreek, adding in some fennel may relieve those symptoms.

Hops

Want an excuse to have a beer? Hops has been rumored to help boost milk production. However, before you get out your chilled mugs, I have some bad news for you. The beer most of us like to drink doesn't have enough hops to have an effect. You have to drink that stuff you can almost chew, like those dark German beers, to show a possible positive effect. I know many of you have probably heard that drinking Guinness is good for milk production (which is why I'm including hops in this list) – this is why. Unfortunately, the effect on milk production doesn't outweigh the negative effects of drinking alcohol, so if you really want to have a beer, drink one you like and stick to just one (see the section on drinking alcohol). There are many other herbs with greater benefits than hops, so it's better to choose one of those.

Herbs That May Decrease Supply

Reactions to herbs are very individual, so before you completely eliminate an herb you absolutely love, try it and see if it affects your supply. Also, while you may be thrilled to just pump out one ounce of your liquid gold, another mama may have so much she's pumping it out by the gallons. So, some of these herbs can be used to help those women produce less. Therefore, you can take it as it suits you – if you feel like your supply is dwindling, avoid these herbs. If you can barely contain those girls, perhaps drinking some tea or taking some supplements of these herbs may tame them a bit. Just be cautious and don't overdo it. Consult an herbalist or holistic practitioner if you have any questions about these herbs.

This list is by no means exhaustive. I'm just listing a few herbs that we commonly consume here. There's a more complete list in the resource booklet that comes with this book at **www.heathermichellenutritionist.com/resourcebooklet**. I also want to mention that if you do an online search on *herbs to avoid while breastfeeding*, you will get whole lists of herbs. However, when you dig deeper, you won't really find any conclusive scientific studies on the true effects of these herbs while lactating. As I said before, research studies are expensive, so it may be that studies just weren't done, and what is known is what women have passed on to each other through generations. However, I think it's more of an individual thing – some herbs affect some women's production, but don't bother other women at all. So, keep this in mind when looking at these lists and consider your own situation. If you want to play it safe, avoid them. But don't be too restrictive. Remember, the goal is to make it easy, not cumbersome, because you want to continue giving your baby breast milk, not feel so deprived that you quit. Use some common sense, monitor your production, and see what works best for you.

Peppermint
I've consistently read that peppermint can negatively affect milk supply, so I did some research on it. As with most herbs, the jury is out. Some women swear that just smelling peppermint affects their supply, while it doesn't affect others at all. I read an article from the Tisserand Institute where the author tried to find the answer to this question, but found nothing. He resorted to polling his Facebook audience and still got answers across the board. Keep in mind, there's nothing scientific about this process, but what he did find is that around 30% of the women who responded said they had negative effects from using peppermint, ranging from tea, oil, mints, even chocolate mint ice cream! This just reinforces the answer is – it just depends. If you are sensitive and you see a drop in your supply, stay away from it. If you are fine with it, go for it!

Just to mention, I did find that some people have side effects in large doses that you really only get in supplement form, like heartburn, nausea, and vomiting. If you have consistent reflux, heartburn, or allergies to any components of peppermint (like menthol), it's best to avoid it, regardless of the effect on your supply.

Parsley and Sage
These are two more herbs that are purported to cause a reduction in milk production, but again, there's no real valid research to show that this is true. There have been some weak studies showing women taking these supplements with no adverse

effects on their supply. According to the Drug and Lactation (LactMed) database, some women in Turkey actually use parsley and sage to boost their supply! Another study of 158 women in Iran had half the group taking a supplement with fennel, anise, cumin, black seed, and parsley and the other half taking a placebo. They measured the weight of the babies over a period and there was no significant difference at the end. However, I didn't find much more information about this study than this, so again, it's a question mark.

Parsley is a member of the Apiaceae family, so if you are allergic to carrot, celery, or fennel, you may have a problem with parsley, but if this is the case, you most likely know about it already. There's even less about sage. It generally just gets thrown in there with parsley. If you love parsley and sage, you may not want to eat a bowl of tabbouleh or sage stuffing right off the bat, but you could try it out in small doses and see how it affects your milk production and your baby.

I'm including a link to the LactMed database in the appendix. There you can search for all of the herbs you have questions about to your heart's content. I could go on and on, but you may be interested in different herbs than I listed here and I want to make sure you finish this book, so I kept the detailed list short. In the end, the effects of most of these herbs on lactation are really just unknown, so it will be a trial and error situation for you. Always err on the side of caution and if you are taking any medications or have any health issues, please consult your practitioner first.

I'm not even going to touch on the subject of safe medication, because, as I said, I'm not a doctor. You need to consult with your doctor or even a pharmacist about meds. You can also take a look at the LactMed database if you want to take a quick look at what is said about taking a certain medications while lactating. But when in doubt, contact your doctor.

Chapter 11
Weight Loss – or Gain?

You've heard it: Breastfeeding is the quickest way to drop pounds after birth! Your body burns an extra 300-700 calories per day to produce milk, so those pounds should be melting off in no time, right? Well, for some women, those extra calories burned do help them drop weight, but some women will actually experience a weight gain – yikes! That's not what you bargained for! Plus, it doesn't help that you probably feel like you are starving and want to binge out all the time, not to mention feeling like you need to drink a gallon of water several times a day. Of course, I'm exaggerating about the water, but this is normal, so don't worry. In the first few months, I felt like I was literally starving, just chowing down. My husband would look at me like an alien took over my body! This is because your body needs those extra calories. However, those extra calories are for producing all that milk, not leaving much left over for burning off extra fat.

Not Rockin' Your High School Jeans?

Did you think you would be rockin' your skinny jeans when leaving the hospital? Or at least your normal jeans within a month or so? You see some women back in their pre-pregnancy jeans practically right out of the hospital and it's so frustrating, you just hate her, right? Some women are just lucky like that, but I can tell you that most women don't drop weight right away. Just when you thought you could put those elastic waistbands away, you can't get out of them. Let me tell you, girlfriend, I was wearing maternity clothes for six months postpartum! It was really around that nine to ten-month mark before I was back to pre-pregnancy weight – it was nine up, nine down for me, and I gained a normal 30 pounds with both of my pregnancies, so I didn't have a long way to go. It really just takes time.

When my son was around 6 weeks old, we had to travel for a wedding. My boobs were huge, the rest of me felt huge too. I had to buy a new dress that would fit this very voluptuous body I was sporting. At the wedding, I was surrounded by these young, thin girls, all svelte and perfect. Talk about hitting my self-esteem! I remember really feeling like crap about myself. The point of telling you this story is that it's normal not to be back to your pre-pregnancy self for a while and it's normal to have these feelings. Just hang in there and focus on your most important task right now – providing your baby with the best nutrition you can. Believe me, this time of breastfeeding will pass in a blink of an eye and after the fact, you will only wish it lasted longer.

Why the Weight isn't Melting Off – Nerd Out Section

I know, this isn't a sexy topic (well, for me it is because I'm a nerd and I love this shit), but for those of you who are nerdy like me or just plain curious, I thought to mention a couple of biochemical reasons why you aren't dropping weight the way you think you should. These aren't meant to be excuses (like, I'm overweight because… and just let yourself go), but perhaps you can be a bit more forgiving and not so hard on yourself if you aren't back to your pre-pregnancy weight as quickly as you'd like.

Ghrelin and Leptin

Some of you may have heard these names before; they were all over the news for a while. Ghrelin is the hunger hormone and leptin is the satiety hormone. So basically, when your body secretes ghrelin, you feel hungry and when it secretes leptin, you feel full. We want more leptin, right? Well, when you have a little one at home, you're probably not getting much sleep at night. I'm sorry to tell you that lack of sleep can boost ghrelin levels (making you feel hungry) and drops leptin, so you don't feel satisfied. I can hear you saying to yourself, *ah, now I know why I'm like a bottomless pit these days*! And now you know why you always hear that lack of sleep causes weight gain. Cool, huh?

You are probably saying, *yeah, cool, but not so cool that I can't get around the lack of sleep right now and I don't want to keep feeling like I can eat an elephant!* No fear, there's a way around this, not a miracle cure, but it will help. It has to do with what you are putting in your mouth. I will explain more about this later when I talk about the best diet for you right now, so keep reading!

Endocannabinoid System
This is relatively new research, so there's not much about it yet (as of this writing), but it's basically like it sounds – it affects the same system as the one that gives you the munchies when you smoke pot. It was found that lack of sleep caused a boost in endocannabinoid levels, causing hedonic, or pleasure, eating. Basically, you grab comfort food, like chips and donuts, with decreased resistance to chow down on them. To make matters worse, a more recent study found that this same system plays a role in your olfactory system, the one that is connected to what you smell, shifting food choices towards – you guessed it, high calorie, high-fat foods. Does this sound like you? Now you know why you may be reaching for that junk food! If you had a rough night, detour far away from Cinnabon; you may not be able to resist the smell wafting from it!

Prolactin
This hormone is necessary to stimulate milk production, so you will find it in high levels in lactating women. Prolactin can also be found in high levels in non-lactating women, and even men, for various reasons. Most of the research done on prolactin and weight has been done with these people because they shouldn't have these high levels of the hormone circulating in their blood. For nursing women, it's considered a non-issue because it's supposed to be there, so there's virtually no research on prolactin, lactation and weight. Basically, prolactin can stimulate hunger and affect fat metabolism, as well as overall metabolism (i.e. calorie burning). The reason for this is because you NEED those extra calories to produce milk, so it's Mother Nature's way of saying EAT! If you've tried to cut calories while breastfeeding, I'm sure you've noticed your milk supply also dropped. It's like trying to drive your car with no gas – it just won't work! So, the very hormone that you need to produce milk is actually making you hungry and holding on to some of that fat.

Now, I hesitated to include this one because I don't want you to go freaking out on me, "OMG, hell no, I'm not breastfeeding if it's going to make me hold onto fat!" Hold your horses. First of all, your body actually produces more prolactin while you are pregnant, preparing you for breastfeeding; your levels are lower while breastfeeding. Second, the benefits of breastfeeding for you and your baby far outweigh you holding on to a few extra pounds for a few months. Third, the elevated prolactin levels are temporary and will go back to normal once you wean your child. Fourth, if you eat properly and move, the excess weight will be minimal. Do I need to mention a fifth? I'm only telling you about this so you understand why you may not be dropping weight like you thought you would. This too will end. Focus on the bigger picture!

Stress
You've heard of these hormones: adrenaline and cortisol. You know, these are the stress, or "fight or flight," hormones. What you may not know is that when they are released into the bloodstream, it's their job to release carbohydrates (i.e. glucose) and fats for immediate energy. You know, if a lion is chasing you, you need fuel, quick! Your appetite is suppressed as well because who would be thinking about eating while running for their life? Plus, all your blood and energy are going to the parts of the body needed to run and fight, not the parts needed for digestion. Once you are safe and sound, your adrenaline dissipates, but your cortisol sticks around and it's like, "we need to replenish all that energy we just burned." So, your appetite gets boosted and you want to eat something. However, we aren't exactly running away from lions anymore. Most of the time, we get this reaction while sitting on our asses behind a desk or behind the steering wheel of a car. So, you didn't burn any of that energy your body just made available, and now your body thinks you need to replenish all that energy you didn't actually burn off.

Nowadays, we tend to stay in this fight or flight mode because we don't outrun and hide from what stresses us out in the first place, so there's no relief, causing us to constantly pump out these hormones. This whole situation ends up being a triple whammy: 1) cortisol makes you hungry, 2) you aren't in the mood to make the effort to make a meal or eat a big salad, so you go for convenient, comfort food, like those cookies sitting in the jar on the counter, 3) insulin levels also spike as a result of all this, causing increased fat deposition, particularly right in your belly. I could go on forever about all the bad effects stress has on your health, but let's just suffice it to say that you need to find a way to CHILL OUT! I know,

I've said this several times already, but it's really important. We, as a species, but particularly as women, worry too much about everything. Take a deep breath and think, "Can I do anything about this situation?" If you can, then do it. If you can't, stop worrying about it! It really doesn't do you any good.

I know, you are probably saying, "What does she know? This isn't something you just turn off!" I'm with ya, it's not that easy. However, there are some things you can do to help. Exercise is key and effective in many ways. You've heard of endorphins, our natural "opioids," as I call them. They give you that high when you have a great workout. They also help relieve stress. Even just getting away from what's stressing you out for a short period will be helpful – a stretch, a bathroom break, a walk to the kitchen for a glass of water, can help get you away from the situation and clear your mind. I know when you have a little one, it's not so easy to just get away, but take him along in his stroller. Meet up with a friend. You can even ask a friend if they can take your bouncing bundle of joy for a couple of hours so you can get a break – maybe a much-deserved mani/pedi. Or get a sitter for a date night with hubby. It doesn't have to be for hours – you don't even have to worry about leaving pumped milk. Just a short time can do wonders when you have a little one attached to your breast for what seems like 24/7. Make it happen – you are worth it! If you want more ideas for alleviating stress, get my resource booklet at **www.heathermichellenutritionist.com/resourcebooklet**.

Medication to Boost Supply
Taking medication to boost supply is definitely not your first option, but for some women, like adoptive mothers who want to breastfeed, those wanting to reinitiate supply, or for women whose babies just cannot nurse at the breast and they want to stimulate more supply for pumping, it may be necessary. However, the main mechanism behind these medications is that they stimulate prolactin production, and, as you just learned, prolactin can cause increased hunger. If you are one of these women, your number one objective is to get your milk flowing so that you can feed your baby the best thing you can provide, so don't focus on your weight right now. Before you know it, the breastfeeding will be over, or your flow will be established and you will be able to stop taking the medication, and you will have plenty of time to work on dropping that weight.

The Good News

I know you want to get back to that svelte, pre-pregnancy body you had right away, but really, what's a year in your life to provide the best nutrition you can for your baby? Let me tell you, once your precious one starts getting an opinion of her own, trying to get nutritious foods into her body will be a challenge, so take advantage of this time to get that nutrition in her while she's not talking back or spitting/throwing food at you!

The main thing you need to focus on is WHAT you are eating. I promise you don't have to diet and you will drop some weight, but you have to be reasonable. If you regularly consume sugary drinks (soft drinks, energy drinks, even smoothies made with fruit juices), grab a salted caramel mocha frappuccino on the way to the park, that Cinnabon that smells so amazing, a value meal at Wendy's because you are in a hurry or just don't feel like cooking (you get the picture), you will definitely have trouble dropping weight. Remember, I said breastfeeding burns 500 extra calories a day, not 1000. On the other side of it, you DO need to eat! Over-restricting your caloric intake can cause the problem of decreased supply, not to mention slowing down your metabolism and starting a whole yoyo dieting problem. But I won't get into all that here because this is a book about breastfeeding, not dieting!

The good news is, if you eat from the earth and watch your portion sizes, you will automatically drop weight. Yes, it's really that simple. Maybe I should make it a big secret, package it up in a pill and make billions! But seriously, I've always been a "whole foodie." In my days of weight-loss counseling, I worked with other dietitians and it seemed that we all had our own theories. Mine has always been to eat as whole and close to nature as possible, and eat what you enjoy in portion-controlled amounts. Moderation is key. You have to live, enjoy and not always feel deprived.

The Big Secret

OK, since I love you like a sister, I'm just going to give you the big secret right here: eat whole, real foods, including whole grains, fill half your plate with veggies and stay away from refined sugars (and flours, while you are at it). Be reasonable:

fill up on the good stuff, have small amounts of the not-so-good stuff. Yep, that's it! No magic wand or pill, just common sense. When I say common sense, that also means that you shouldn't be munching out every five minutes, or eating huge amounts of foods either, no matter how healthy the food is. Even though you get to eat more because you are lactating, you don't get unlimited get-out-of-jail-free cards; it has to be within reason. We all know when we are doing things we shouldn't, this is no different. Just like when you are speeding down the highway, you take your chances with the consequences of getting caught and getting a ticket. However, in that case, you may not actually get caught and thus not get a ticket. However, in the case of eating a bunch of junk, you are guaranteed to get caught because you can't fool your body! You can sidestep the consequences when you "break the law" sometimes, but if it's consistent and you are eating crap more often than you are eating the way you should, your get-out-of-jail-free cards will be voided.

This doesn't mean that you have to make absolutely everything from scratch. I know that's not reasonable for most, especially with a wee one in the house. Yes, you can buy a snack bar or other convenience foods, but when you read the label, make sure it contains ingredients you would have in your own kitchen (or could easily buy), and that one of the first couple ingredients isn't sugar or a derivative. You need the calories right now to make milk, so go ahead and eat, because you will be hungry. Just make sure WHAT you are eating is conducive to good health. Of course, you can have that cookies and cream cone dipped in Oreo crumbs once in a while, but make sure it's just a treat, not a regular thing.

Simple right? Then why do so many people have such a hard time? There are so many components that go into this, but it's mostly about our mindset and how we've been programmed from young. What were you served at home growing up? Were you part of the "you have to clean your plate" group? Were you given a treat to make you feel better when you scraped your knee or were disappointed by something? Did your parents always have sweet treats around the house? Did you run through McDonald's drive-thru as a regular thing? This can go on and on, but the thing to remember here is that it's no one's fault and no one is to blame. Most parents do the best they can and most of these things they did with you, their parents did with them. The other side of this is that we just don't know how to prepare different foods, and most of us take the path of least resistance, especially when juggling so many things on our (non-literal) plates. Stay tuned for my next book, which will be on this very topic!

The way to change your eating and lifestyle habits is to be aware, educate yourself, have the desire to do it, and start making the change! You can teach an old dog new tricks, so you, young whippersnapper, can learn new tricks too!

I want to mention that I know that there are a few diets out there right now that say that grains are bad and that we should stay away from them. I agree that we should stay away from processed grains, but I do advocate whole grains because they contain most of the nutrients your body needs and they will help you feel full. However, you have to eat them whole, with the bran and germ intact (the two components of the grain that are the most nutrient-rich and that are removed in processing). Besides, do you think it's realistic to go through your whole life never eating grains again (that includes bread, pasta, pancakes and so much more!)? I could write a whole book about grains (hey, maybe I will!), but let's suffice it to say that unless you have issues, like an autoimmune disease that affects your gut or epilepsy, you should be fine. So yes, there are select groups of people who would do better without any grains, but they are not as prevalent as the trends may lead you to believe. If you are in doubt about your personal situation, contact your doctor.

Remember our conversation about ghrelin and leptin? You want to boost leptin levels, the hormone that makes you feel full, right? Well, eating as I outlined above will do just that. Increasing your fiber intake by consuming foods like whole grains and beans will help boost leptin. While you are at it, boosting intake of these foods, and lowering intake of those white flours and white sugar, will also help because processed grains and sugars mess around with your insulin "system," which in turn messes with the positive effects of leptin that you want. Also, lowering triglycerides, a type of fat, will help to boost leptin, and you do this by eating as I told you – lots of veggies, whole grains, cutting out the sugars (especially those sugary drinks), and consuming healthy fats, like avocado or olives and their oils, as well as nuts and seeds. I extremely simplified this process here, but hopefully, you get my drift.

Let's not forget the importance of exercise - get out there and move! Put your baby in a stroller and take a walk. Meet up with a girlfriend or get your significant other out there. God knows you need adult conversation and quality time with loved ones. If you are able, get some HIIT (high-intensity interval training) workouts a couple of times a week. You will be amazed at how your body can actually get back to "normal." Well, I have to be honest and tell you it will be a new normal because it just doesn't go exactly back to where it was. My waist never went back, but my hips did and I really didn't think it would happen after my second. Be patient and forgiving. It will come!

Part V
After One Year

Your baby has hit one year! Where did the time go? Hopefully, you were able to make it this far breastfeeding your baby. If you did, congratulations! If you didn't, be proud of what you were able to provide for your preciousness. After one year, your baby can handle almost all normal food and can drink regular milk, so providing meals for your baby gets a lot easier. There are a couple of things I want to mention, plus reoccurring topics from other women, that I would like to share with you.

Chapter 12
Your Baby is a Year Old! What's Next?

You got through the first year and are now at the point where you have to make a decision – continue breastfeeding or start giving regular (whole) milk. This is really a personal choice. The World Health Organization recommends breast-feeding for two years, but if you choose, you can stop. Nutritionally, breast milk is better than cow – cow milk proteins are difficult to digest, even for some adults to digest! But if you are really done, then give yourself a pat on the back for making it to a year and start providing your baby with nutritious meals full of the foods I mentioned in "The Big Secret." I highly recommend the book, "Super Baby Food," by Ruth Yaron. You should actually start using this book the moment you start giving your baby solids, but she has tips, recipes, and info beyond food in this book that you will find very helpful.

Which type of Milk is Best?

Regarding milk, if you choose to give your baby milk from an animal besides yourself, I recommend goat or sheep milk. Nutritionally and palatability speaking, sheep milk has an excellent profile. However, sheep are known to be very difficult to milk, so you will be hard-pressed to find any. If you are fortunate enough to find a farmer who will sell you sheep milk, great!

The proteins in these kinds of milk are smaller and much more digestible than that from a cow. Think about it, cow babies eventually grow to be around 1500 pounds when they are adults, so the nutrient needs of a calf are much different than that of a human baby. Goats and sheep end up being anywhere between 80 to 280 pounds (depending on the type), which is much more closely related to human adult weights.

Besides the size issue, there are nutritional benefits in goat milk that you don't find in cow milk. Cow milk is full of lactose, which many cannot tolerate, and it is known to be acidic and allergenic. The main offending protein in cow milk that's the root cause of many allergies is alpha-s1-casein. Goat milk is the closest to human milk in structure. It has very little or almost no alpha-s1-casein, which is one reason why people who cannot tolerate cow milk do just fine with goat milk (around 40% of people who have cow milk allergies can drink goat milk with no ill effects). Goat milk has smaller fat globules than cow, with a high amount of medium-chain fatty acids, making it more digestible. There are more benefits with goat milk over cow, but I won't include an exhaustive list here. If you want more information, check out my resource booklet at: **www.heathermichellenutritionist.com/resourcebooklet**.

The only downside to goat milk is that after the commercial pasteurization process, it can have that gamey flavor which causes most to turn their nose up to it. Your baby won't really know the difference and will most likely drink it just fine (mine did!), so go ahead and buy it in the store. However, if you can get fresh goat milk, there won't be any of that gamey taste at all. I know you are thinking that raw milk will surely make your baby sick. I don't want to tell you to give raw milk to your baby, he happens to get sick, and then you point your finger at me that I told you to do it, so pasteurize the milk yourself. Basically, you bring your milk to a temperature of 161° F for 15 seconds, then pour it into containers and put them into an ice bath immediately. This method has the least effect on flavor and it will still be much fresher than store-bought.

I'm suggesting goat milk, rather than cow, for your one+-year-olds who have no apparent allergies. If your child has, or appears to have, a true cow milk allergy, please contact your doctor before trying goat milk.

No Periods Yet?

Some women get their period almost right after giving birth (so sorry, girlfriend!). Others, like me, had to completely stop breastfeeding altogether to get a period. Women are asking this question all the time – when will their period start again? There's no real answer; everyone is different. Just watch out, because you can ovulate without knowing and get pregnant before you even have a cycle again!

It seemed no matter how infrequently I was feeding (I got down to only one feeding a day), still no period. For some of you, this is no problem and actually very welcome, but others, like me, may want to get pregnant again. This is really the only reason I stopped breastfeeding my son at 13 months. It was really just perfect – he was only feeding morning and evening, so I didn't have to worry about wearing something boob-accessible, and he was sleeping through the night. I definitely could have gone two years like that. However, it took me a while to get pregnant with him and I wasn't getting any younger, so I really wanted to get back on the fertile bandwagon again.

If this is you, you may decide to stop at this point to start on the next baby. If you are loving having no periods, then keep going, baby! Take advantage of not getting the monthly visit of hell and enjoy those breastfeeding moments with your baby.

Still Not Sleeping Through the Night?

There are many reasons why babies don't sleep through the night, but since this is a book on breastfeeding, I will stick to this topic.

Maybe you were one of those moms who stuck to her guns and you taught your baby to sleep on her own; no falling asleep on the breast, or when baby wakes up at night you let her self-soothe (taking a quick check to make sure all is OK and let her be). If you are one of those moms, then great for you! That means this section most likely doesn't apply to you because your baby is sleeping through the night.

However, if you are like me where you were just too tired to deal with a crying baby in the middle of the night and stuck her on the breast when she woke up, you may just be able to relate. Some of you may be waving your finger back and forth at me, but remember when I told you I went with my instincts? I didn't always do the perfect thing, and I'll tell you right now, missy, you won't either! The things you said you would never do before you had kids, when you watched other people's brats, you find yourself doing to your dismay! But once you are a parent, you learn not to ever judge others again because everyone has the best intentions, and sometimes, it's just not a perfect world. But, I digress.

So, yes, when my daughter woke up at night, I would stick her on the breast so she would shut up and I could get some sleep. Funny enough, I pretty much did the same thing with my son and by one year, he was sleeping through the night on his own. So, it just goes to show you that all babies are different! Perhaps that's why I gave the breast at night again when I had my daughter – it went so perfect the first time! But after a year, then 13 months, then 14, and so on, she kept waking up for the breast. I really became a pacifier. I just couldn't take it anymore, so by 17 months, I had to stop. Lucky for me, I had the perfect opportunity because I planned a cruise for my 40th birthday and was able to escape for 10 days – the perfect amount of time to let my milk run dry, and for her to get adjusted to not having the breast anymore. By the time I got back, it was done – and as I said before, she went right from the breast to a cup, no bottle for her! I did bring my little hand pump with me to relieve some pressure in my breasts, but I hardly had to use it at all.

My advice here is that all babies are different. Some will eventually sleep through the night, even while breastfeeding, and some will wake you up every night indefinitely. It's your call when you decide that it's enough!

Grabbing the Boob in Public

As you get past the first year and you are still breastfeeding in public, you will be getting looks from people. Some may be encouraging, but you will find those looks like, "OMG! She's STILL breastfeeding?" This will probably come more frequently as your baby, now toddler, gets a bit older, like closer to two years old. Just remember, it's YOUR decision.

There's also that point where your little one will start pulling on your shirt and going for your boob in public. I never got to that point with mine, since I didn't get past one and a half years, but I have seen this many times, even with my own girlfriends. We are trying to have a conversation and her toddler comes to pull up her shirt. Most of the time, my girlfriend does not want this and is trying to get her child to go play. For me, this was definitely a big no-no; I always had it in my mind that I would not let my child do that. However, that's me. You may not mind this and it's your prerogative to do as you wish. You know what's right for you!

Epilogue

Before having kids, people would tell me, "your life will never be the same again," or "your life will change completely." I would think to myself, "No way, I'm not going to let this change my life!" Well, of course, it did. I never slept the same way again, you will never react the same when you hear any kid, anywhere, yelling "MOM," even the people you hang around with won't be the same (yes, it's true, you end up hanging around people who have kids that your kids want to hang around with). However, this is one of the most amazing times of your life. You, as a woman, have the opportunity to have the experience to feel something growing inside of you, and the ability to provide nourishment, plus an amazing bonding experience, with this bundle of love and joy. You get to be the object of unconditional admiration from your baby – you are the one she goes to for comfort, uncertainty, when afraid, when happy about something - everything. It may seem exhausting to be the end-all, be-all for another being, but believe me when I tell you, it ends in a blink of an eye and you wish you could get it back. Take this time to savor the moments, don't feel like you have to rush to stop breastfeeding, or rush to do anything. Now that I have teenagers, I understand why grandparents love their grandchildren so much – they get to do it all over again!

Now that you've read through this book, I hope you're convinced about making the decision to breastfeed your baby. You understand the reasons why breast is best and have created the mindset to make it happen! You've formed your support team, filled in your baby registry with all of the essentials, and even started browsing for nursing tops. While we are creating this image, let's go further! You've cut out at least one, if not two sugary beverages a day, started incorporating whole grains in your diet (like brown rice, instead of white), and are loading up your shopping cart (and your plate) with fresh fruits and vegetables! Remember, big changes don't happen overnight, so take small steps and praise yourself for every step in the right direction. Most importantly, express gratitude every day. Be grateful that you can get pregnant and have a baby in the first place. Be grateful for a healthy baby. Be grateful for your ability to breastfeed your baby. Be grateful for your support team around you. If things don't turn out quite as you plan, be grateful for the opportunity to share in the love of another being in a way you never thought you could. Because no matter what happens, that love is priceless and you will always have it, no matter what.

I do want to mention that I am sensitive to the fact that some women just have a hard time breastfeeding and/or just dealing with having a newborn, and women who are dealing with postpartum depression have an additional challenge. I didn't mention this before because I don't want to create a reason for an excuse, but in the end, there are various reasons why, try as you might, breastfeeding just doesn't work for you. After reading this book, I know you will have tried everything and gotten all of the support you could possibly get, but for one reason or another, it just didn't happen. Thankfully, we do have an alternative for babies that's formulated to be as close to the breast as possible. It doesn't replace breast milk by a long shot, but it's a far cry from giving babies powdered milk (i.e. Carnation babies) or milk straight from the cow like moms had to do in the old days. So, focus your energy on enjoying your baby, and let go of any guilty feelings you may have for not being able to breastfeed. It's more important that your baby gets the best mama he can get than suboptimal energy from you because you are focused on what you couldn't provide. There's so much more to mothering and nurturing your baby than just breastfeeding, so focus on what you CAN provide. You've got this, Mama!

I truly hope that you enjoyed reading this book, that it was informative, that you learned a lot that will help you in your breastfeeding journey, and that you also got a good laugh along the way! If I accomplished that, then my purpose here has been fulfilled. But your journey as a woman through the stages of life will continue, and I won't leave you hanging, girlfriend! I will be there for you when you have kids in school, with all their activities, you being mom taxi, wife, household manager, and career woman, you must still take care of your own health in the process. How the hell do you do that? Stick with me and I'll give you my girlfriend to girlfriend best!

Resources

Benefits of Breastfeeding on Infant Health

Immunological Effects of Human Milk Oligosaccharides
https://www.frontiersin.org/articles/10.3389/fped.2018.00190/full

Breastfeeding Tied to Reduced Risk of Serious Infant Infections
https://www.medscape.com/viewarticle/939727

https://consumer.healthday.com/b-11-10-breastfeeding-boosts-babys-mental-health-2648792435.html

https://www.healio.com/news/primary-care/20201112/exclusive-breastfeeding-results-in-drastic-reduction-of-pediatric-dental-disease

https://www.foodandnutritionjournal.org/volume2number2/importance-of-exclusive-breastfeeding-and-complementary-feeding-among-infants/

Food Restrictions

https://www.evenflofeeding.com/education/feeding-101/foods-to-avoid-while-breastfeeding

Maternal Food Restrictions During Breastfeeding

https://www.ncbi.nlm.nih.gov/pmc/articles/PMC5383635/

https://www.healthline.com/health/parenting/breastfeeding-made-me-gain-weight#4.-Hormones,-schmormones

https://consumer.healthday.com/b-3-9-should-breastfeeding-women-avoid-certain-foods-if-baby-has-an-allergy-2650896790.html

Returning to Work

https://www.womenshealth.gov/breastfeeding/breastfeeding-home-work-and-public/breastfeeding-and-going-back-work

https://familydoctor.org/breastfeeding-returning-to-work/

https://www.dol.gov/agencies/whd/fact-sheets/73-flsa-break-time-nursing-mothers

https://www.dol.gov/agencies/whd/nursing-mothers/faq

https://www.drjaygordon.com/blog-detail/nursing-and-working-my-secrets

Pumping and Storing Expressed Milk

https://www.cdc.gov/breastfeeding/recommendations/handling_breastmilk.htm

https://www.cdc.gov/breastfeeding/recommendations/faq.html#expressed

https://www.cdc.gov/healthywater/hygiene/healthychildcare/infantfeeding/breastpump.html

https://www.verywellfamily.com/can-you-mix-fresh-and-previously-collected-breast-milk-431750

https://pregnant.sg/articles/handling-frozen-breast-milk/

Human Milk Storage Guidelines PDF
https://www.cdc.gov/breastfeeding/pdf/HumanMilk-en-508.pdf

Weight Gain

Increased Body Weight Associated with Prolactin Secreting Pituitary Adenomas: Weight Loss with Normalization of Prolactin Levels
https://pubmed.ncbi.nlm.nih.gov/9666865/

https://parenting.firstcry.com/articles/gaining-weight-after-stopping-breastfeeding-is-it-common/

https://www.popsugar.com/family/How-Breastfeeding-Can-Make-You-Gain-Weight-37837572

https://www.webmd.com/fitness-exercise/features/weight-gain-linked-to-stress#1

A Single Night of Sleep Deprivation Increases Ghrelin Levels and Feelings of Hunger in Normal-Weight Healthy Men
https://pubmed.ncbi.nlm.nih.gov/18564298/

https://www.webmd.com/diet/foods-to-boost-leptin#2

https://consumerscompanion.com/how-to-increase-leptin-and-decrease-ghrelin/

https://leptin-resistance.com/leptin-and-insulin-resistance/

https://www.healthline.com/health/parenting/how-many-ounces-do-newborns-need-to-eat#formulafed

https://www.nih.gov/news-events/nih-research-matters/molecular-ties-between-lack-sleep-weight-gain

Sleep Restriction Enhances the Daily Rhythm of Circulating Levels of Endocannabinoid 2-Arachidonoylglycerol https://pubmed.ncbi.nlm.nih.gov/26612385/

Olfactory Connectivity Mediates Sleep-Dependent Food Choices in Humans
https://elifesciences.org/articles/49053

General Nutrition Info

https://www.momjunction.com/articles/flaxseed-breastfeeding-lactation-safety-benefits_00630869/

https://fdc.nal.usda.gov/fdc-app.html#/food-details/169414/nutrients

Energy and Protein Requirements During Lactation
https://pubmed.ncbi.nlm.nih.gov/9240917/

https://www.netmeds.com/health-library/post/protein-needs-during-pregnancy-and-lactation/

https://www.nrv.gov.au/nutrients/waters

Nutrition for Pregnant and Lactating Women: The Latest Recommendations from the Dietary Guidelines for Americans 2020-2025 and Practice Implications
https://journals.sagepub.com/doi/10.1177/15598276211004082

https://www.acog.org/womens-health/experts-and-stories/ask-acog/how-much-coffee-can-i-drink-while-pregnant

https://nutritiondata.self.com/facts/nut-and-seed-products/3115/2

Dietary Reference Intakes (DRI's): Vitamins
https://www.ncbi.nlm.nih.gov/books/NBK56068/table/summarytables.t2/?report=objectonly

Dietary Reference Intakes (DRI's): Elements (minerals)
https://www.ncbi.nlm.nih.gov/books/NBK545442/table/appJ_tab3/?report=objectonly

https://ods.od.nih.gov/HealthInformation/Dietary_Reference_Intakes.aspx

https://www.healthline.com/nutrition/breastfeeding-diet-101#breast-milk-basics

Maternal Versus Infant Vitamin D Supplementation During Lactation: A Randomized Controlled Trial
https://www.ncbi.nlm.nih.gov/pmc/articles/PMC4586731/

https://americanpregnancy.org/healthy-pregnancy/pregnancy-health-wellness/vitamin-d-and-pregnancy-4915/

https://americanpregnancy.org/healthy-pregnancy/breastfeeding/postnatal-vitamins-while-breastfeeding-15365/

Calcium Intakes and Bone Densities of Lactating Women and Breast-fed Infants in The Gambia
https://pubmed.ncbi.nlm.nih.gov/7832054/

Maternal Calcium Requirements During Pregnancy and Lactation
https://pubmed.ncbi.nlm.nih.gov/8304285/

Calcium in Pregnancy and Lactation
https://pubmed.ncbi.nlm.nih.gov/10940334/

https://ods.od.nih.gov/factsheets/Calcium-HealthProfessional/

https://www.cambridge.org/core/journals/proceedings-of-the-nutrition-society/article/human-milk-maternal-dietary-lipids-and-infant-development/FD36C50F12B5D28EE9A6559EA1AC4E9D

https://journals.lww.com/jpgn/Fulltext/2009/03001/Omega_3_Fatty_Acids_and_Neural_Development_to_2.4.aspx

Omega-3 Fatty Acids and Neural Development to 2 Years of Age: Do We Know Enough for Dietary Recommendations?
https://pubmed.ncbi.nlm.nih.gov/19214053/

http://www.dhaomega3.org/FAQ/Is-there-a-Tolerable-Upper-Limit-for-Omega-3-intake-in-adults

https://www.grassrootshealth.net/blog/much-epa-dha-omega-3-supplement/

https://ods.od.nih.gov/factsheets/Omega3FattyAcids-HealthProfessional/

Breast milk DHA Levels May Increase After Informing Women: A Community-based Cohort Study from South Dakota USA
https://www.ncbi.nlm.nih.gov/pmc/articles/PMC5273852/

https://www.nutritionvalue.org/Coconut_water%2C_unsweetened_nutritional_value.html?size=1+coconut+yields+%3D+206+g

https://coconuthandbook.tetrapak.com/chapter/chemistry-coconut-water

Herbs

A Review of Herbal and Pharmaceutical Galactagogues for Breastfeeding
https://www.ncbi.nlm.nih.gov/pmc/articles/PMC5158159/

https://www.uspharmacist.com/article/nonprescription-products-for-the-pregnant-and-breast-feeding-patient

https://www.drjaygordon.com/blog-detail/mothers-milk-how-to-increase-your-supply

https://herblore.com/overviews/list-of-galactagogues-herbs-that-increase-breastmilk-production

https://kellymom.com/bf/got-milk/herbs_to_avoid/

https://milkdust.com/fenugreek-the-good-and-bad-for-breastfeeding-and-milk-supply/

https://herblore.com/overviews/moringa-info

https://www.mamanatural.com/fenugreek/

Anti-inflammatory Activity of Fenugreek Seed Petroleum Ether Extract
https://www.ncbi.nlm.nih.gov/pmc/articles/PMC4980935/

Drugs and Lactation Database (LactMed)
https://www.ncbi.nlm.nih.gov/books/NBK501922/?report=classic

The Effect of Galactagogue Herbal Tea on Breast milk Production and Short-term Catch-up of Birth Weight in the First Week of Life
https://pubmed.ncbi.nlm.nih.gov/21261516/

https://healthjade.com/peppermint-tea/

https://tisserandinstitute.org/peppermint-and-breastfeeding-results-of-poll/

https://www.drugs.com/breastfeeding/aloe.html https://www.drugs.com/breastfeeding/parsley.html

Parsley
https://pubmed.ncbi.nlm.nih.gov/30000940/

https://kellymom.com/bf/can-i-breastfeed/herbs/herbal-ref/

Goat vs Cow Milk

https://calmerme.com/cow-versus-goat-versus-sheep-milk-comparison/

https://www.weedemandreap.com/milk-showdown-cow-sheep-goat/

Protein Digestion and Quality of Goat and Cow Milk Infant Formula and Human Milk Under Simulated Infant Conditions
https://www.ncbi.nlm.nih.gov/pmc/articles/PMC5704675/

http://www.everything-goat-milk.com/protein-in-milk.html

Comparative Protein Composition Analysis of Goat Milk Produced by Alpine

and Saanen Breeds in Northeastern Brazil and Related Antibacterial Activities
https://www.ncbi.nlm.nih.gov/pmc/articles/PMC3968165/

https://www.nutritionadvance.com/goat-milk-vs-cow-milk/

https://www.wikihow.com/Pasteurize-Milk

Various Topics

https://pleaseibu.com/baby-stories/things-i-wished-people-told-me-about-breastfeeding/

https://www.newhealthadvisor.org/Breastfeeding-After-C-Section.html
https://themommydaily.com/newborns-not-eating/

https://wicbreastfeeding.fns.usda.gov/overcome

https://www.healthline.com/health/parenting/lecithin-breast-feeding#What-Are-the-Benefits

https://www.infantrisk.com/content/breastfeeding-after-breast-augmentation

http://www.med.umich.edu/1libr/Gyn/Lactation/BreastfeedingAfterBreastImplants.pdf

https://kellymom.com/bf/got-milk/supply-worries/fast-letdown/

https://www.mayoclinic.org/diseases-conditions/mastitis/symptoms-causes/syc-20374829

https://www.healthyandnaturalworld.com/sore-nipples/

https://www.laviemom.com/blogs/resources/how-to-travel-while-breastfeeding

https://livingwithlowmilksupply.com/things-that-cause-your-milk-supply-suddenly-dropped https://www.theenergyblueprint.com/fatigue-causes-and-how-to-fix-fatigue/

Caffeine and the Central Nervous System: mechanisms of action, biochemical, metabolic and psychostimulant effects
https://pubmed.ncbi.nlm.nih.gov/1356551/

Estimates of Ethanol Exposure in Children from Food not Labeled as Alcohol-Containing
https://www.ncbi.nlm.nih.gov/pmc/articles/PMC5421578/

https://www.cdc.gov/breastfeeding/breastfeeding-special-circumstances/vaccinations-medications-drugs/alcohol.html

Episode 62 Alcohol and Lactation: A Reassuring Look at the Numbers
https://www.milkminutepodcast.com/learn/

Helpful Resources

Drugs and Lactation (LactMed) Database
https://www.ncbi.nlm.nih.gov/books/NBK501922/?report=classic

Breaktime for Nursing Mothers under the Fair Labor Standards Act
https://www.dol.gov/agencies/whd/fact-sheets/73-flsa-break-time-nursing-mothers

Breaktime for Working Mothers (Laws according to the Affordable Care Act)
https://www.dol.gov/agencies/whd/nursing-mothers/faq

Workplace lactation laws by state https://www.pregnantatwork.org/workplace-lactation-laws

WIC breastfeeding support
https://wicbreastfeeding.fns.usda.gov/

La Leche League International
https://www.llli.org/

Breast pumps and supplies through insurance
https://aeroflowbreastpumps.com/qualify-through-insurance

How to find the Right Breast Pump Flange Size
https://www.drbrownsbaby.com/how-to-find-the-right-breast-pump-flange-size/

Dietary Reference Intakes (DRI's): Vitamins
https://www.ncbi.nlm.nih.gov/books/NBK56068/table/summarytables.t2/?report=objectonly

Dietary Reference Intakes (DRI's): Elements (minerals)
https://www.ncbi.nlm.nih.gov/books/NBK545442/table/appJ_tab3/?report=objectonly

Author Note

Thank you so much for reading my book! Believe it or not, this book was actually a few years in the making. One day, the idea hit me like a comet falling from the sky, so I jotted down a few notes and then just sat on it. It took me a long time to take action, so much so that I felt like I missed the opportunity to write this book. Around the beginning of 2020, right after the whole Coronavirus pandemic, the idea hit me in the head again and I said to myself, don't be a dumbass, sit yourself down and write this book!

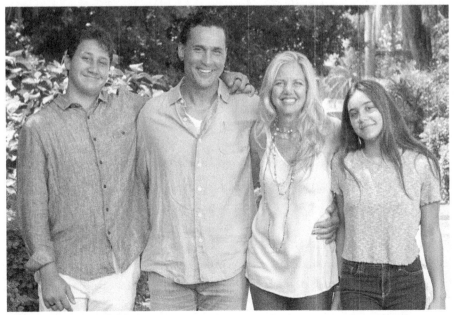

Me with my hubby and the two monsters

During the writing process, I had to get out of my own way, tossing aside feelings of self-doubt, focusing on the women I could help. I had a successful breastfeeding journey, much of which I chalked up to preparing and educating myself before I gave birth. If I could give these same tools to other women, I was sure I could help them too!

Besides getting out of my head, it was also quite a juggle taking time to write and self-publish a book while balancing the needs of two teenagers, a husband and running other businesses (and let's not forget taking care of myself!). If you are already a mom, you know about the pull you get from all directions! If you are a new mom or mom-to-be, you will find out soon enough!

Receiving validation from readers has inspired me to put myself out there in the limelight. From veteran moms telling me they wish they had a book like this when starting out in the breastfeeding process, to women who haven't started on that journey yet but were motivated to breastfeed (even if they weren't planning to) after reading my book, their feedback made all of the sacrifice well worth it!

As I researched content for the book, I read and listened to many comments from women who breastfed their babies, from pains, frustrations and uncertainties, to general questions they had about "how to XYZ." As I read those comments and saw a trend in what was being asked, I would think, I have to include that in my book! So, the 20-30 page little booklet I planned to write turned into a 100+ page book. At the same time, I really wanted to keep the book short and doable for moms and moms-to-be because we are all so busy and may feel intimidated by the idea of having to sit down to read a thick book. I believe the content is so valuable that I wanted to write something you would feel is doable. Personally, when I see a thin book with around 100 pages, I figure I can get that read within a couple of hours and am more likely to read it. With that, there are things that got left out, so the book definitely isn't all encompassing, but the idea is to get you going on your breastfeeding journey by setting out with the right mindset and searching for help from the appropriate professionals along the way.

If you loved the book, either it helped you be successful or you feel like it would have helped you if you had it when you were in that phase, please help get the information in the hands of other women who would benefit from it. If you are willing to write me a review, I would be so appreciative! Reviews help others find my book by getting it at the top of the search page, and make readers more likely to want to read it (I think we all look at reviews when purchasing something nowadays). I also read all of my reviews because I believe your feedback very important. This helps me improve my content so my future books will be even better at helping you, my readers!

Writing this book has been a learning process for me, in more ways than one. I think one of the main things I got out of it is that I can accomplish what I set my mind to, as long as I stay persistent, patient and forgiving with myself, focus on my goals and get the job done! It's this same philosophy that will help all of us be successful in breastfeeding, in our career, and in everything in life. Achieving this goal has helped me aspire to continue writing books to help women in their health and wellness goals, so stay tuned for my next book, which will be about how we can achieve our nutrition and fitness goals by working on our mindset.

We are all working towards achieving better health and wellness, sometimes we just get stuck and need a little nudge. Follow me for the latest info in my blogs, social media posts, and sign up for my bi-monthly newsletters at: **www.heathermichellenutritionist.com**.

Facebook: Heather Michelle Nutritionist

Instagram: @heathermichellenutritionist

About the Author

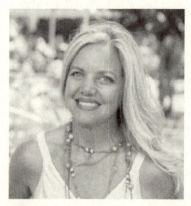

Heather Michelle de Paulo is registered dietitian, a mother of two teens, entrepreneur, household chef and baker, mom taxi and, like so many women, the glue that holds everything together. She is passionate about helping women make their health a priority across the mom-life journey. She started her career working in the clinical setting, as well as helping HIV/AIDS patients and those recovering from drug and alcohol abuse. She later worked in weight loss and medical nutrition therapy, and has served as a dietitian and research coordinator for numerous pharmaceutical and nutraceutical research studies. After becoming a mom, she identified the need to help other moms understand that their own health has to be a priority, empowering them to believe it's doable by taking quick, actionable steps to reach their goals, using a lifestyle approach. Heather is a huge breastfeeding advocate, having exclusively breastfed both of her babies, and has been passionate about helping her friends and all women overcome challenges they may have while breastfeeding their own babies. She currently lives on the island of Curaçao, with her husband, her two teenage monsters, and three dogs.

If you would like to receive Heather's research, recipes and advice on a regular basis, you can subscribe to her newsletter at **www.heathermichellenutritionist.com**.

Made in the USA
Las Vegas, NV
04 November 2021